ENDING THE HIV EPIDEMIC

COMMUNITY STRATEGIES
IN DISEASE PREVENTION
AND HEALTH PROMOTION

ENDING THE HIV EPIDEMIC

COMMUNITY STRATEGIES IN DISEASE PREVENTION AND HEALTH PROMOTION

Edited by Steven Petrow
with Pat Franks and Timothy R. Wolfred

San Francisco AIDS Foundation
Institute for Health Policy Studies
and
Center for AIDS Prevention Studies
University of California, San Francisco

Network Publications, a division of ETR Associates
Santa Cruz, California
1990

Development of this book was assisted by a grant from The Robert Wood Johnson Foundation and grant MH42459 from the National Institute of Mental Health. The opinions, conclusions and proposals in the text are those of the authors and do not necessarily represent those of The Robert Wood Johnson Foundation; the National Institute of Mental Health; the Institute for Health Policy Studies and the Center for AIDS Prevention Studies, University of California, San Francisco; the San Francisco AIDS Foundation; or any other agency or institution associated with the development of the text.

Printed in the United States of America
10 9 8 7 6 5 4 3 2 1

Cover design: Julia Chiapella

Title No. 550 (hardbound)
Title No. 345 (softbound)

Library of Congress Cataloging-in-Publication Data
Ending the HIV epidemic : community strategies in disease prevention and health
    promotion / edited by Steven Petrow, with Pat Franks and Timothy R. Wolfred.
        p. cm.
    ISBN 1-56071-033-0
        1. AIDS (Disease)—Prevention. 2. AIDS (Disease)—California—San Francisco—Prevention. 3. Health education. I. Petrow, Steven. II. Franks, Pat. III. Wolfred, Timothy R.
        [DNLM: 1. Acquired Immunodeficiency Syndrome—epidemiology—San Francisco. 2. Acquired Immunodeficiency Syndrome—prevention & control—San Francisco. 3. Community Health Services—San Francisco. 4. Disease Outbreaks—prevention & control—San Francisco. 5. Health Promotion—San Francisco.]
    RA644.A25E53 1990
    614.5'993—dc20
    DNLM/DLC   90-6384
    for Library of Congress   CIP

This book is dedicated to Sam B. Puckett (1937-1988). Sam was a longtime San Franciscan, a lawyer, a Southern gentleman, a curmudgeon, a community activist, a gay man and an innovator in AIDS prevention. Cofounder of the STOP AIDS Project, Sam was convinced from the start that AIDS prevention was not really a "health education issue" but a social marketing one, an issue centered on understanding community norms and values. The question he posed for himself and others as we began to write this book was, How do we create new patterns of interaction within the community that support new patterns of behavior and health?

Contents

Foreword

In early 1981, a condition indicative of immune deficiency was seen in a few young men in California and New York. Even as the numbers began to increase, no one could have predicted that by the end of the 1980s, over 100,000 more individuals in the prime of life would be diagnosed with the same problem and well over 60,000 of them would be dead as a result of it.

Today, almost every community is touched by the HIV epidemic, caused by infection with the human immunodeficiency virus. Public health leaders are recognizing that this epidemic is different from other health problems. Because of the relationship of the spread of HIV to sexual behavior, particularly gay male sexual behavior, and illicit drug use activities, those infected and the groups they represent have been stigmatized. Homophobia, racism and irrational fear, leading to discrimination and even violence, have made this disease not only a medical problem, but a social and political one as well.

This means that communities will have to be proactive, to take risks and to learn from the successes and failures of other affected communities. How communities respond will determine how effective we will be in ending this nightmare.

Historically, when faced with a new health crisis, governments have attempted to take control, to determine the nature and scope of the problem and to provide, to the extent possible, the necessary human and financial resources. However, with the advent of AIDS, it became very clear that this new "plague" was unlike those of the past and needed innovative approaches. In order to prevent the spread of HIV infection, different educational and prevention programs were required to convince individuals and groups to change very basic, personal behaviors.

The San Francisco Department of Public Health recognized at the outset that it should serve as a convener and facilitator, bringing together public health leaders, private physicians, researchers, established community groups, people with AIDS, and experts in communication, education and marketing. Once a plan of action was agreed upon, the Department served as the funding source for programs to be implemented, in large part by the gay community, and later by ethnic minority organizations. Working together, although not always in perfect harmony, San Francisco's various agencies and organizations created a response that has served as a model both nationally and worldwide.

Throughout the epidemic, there has been an emphasis on problem solving within the affected communities. The result has been not only more humane and compassionate services, but also more effective care at a lower cost. Also, early in the epidemic, the availability of culturally-sensitive and language-appropriate educational and informational programs may have had an effect on the incredible decline in unsafe sexual behavior among gay men, with a concomitant reduction in new infections, which fell to less than 1 percent in 1987. Unfortunately, there appears to be a relatively small relapse rate among this group, which demonstrates the importance of continued prevention activities for all at-risk populations.

The lessons learned in San Francisco are presented in this book as a case study of a community in action. To end this epidemic, each community must mount an aggressive prevention campaign that never loses sight of the human tragedy of HIV disease. Obviously, no two settings are alike—each is different politically, socially and economically—but most of the HIV prevention strategies discussed in the following chapters can be adapted to the special needs of each particular population.

Most of the authors of *Ending the HIV Epidemic* have participated in the development and implementation of San Francisco's overall prevention effort and are to be credited in large part for its success. They clearly demonstrate that the importance of working together cannot be overestimated. Furthermore, the fact that they write from their own experience and involvement in the process adds to the strength of this book.

Sadly, a number of cities and localities have been—and are being—overwhelmed by this epidemic. Even San Francisco is feeling the crushing pressure of a rapidly increasing caseload, a dwindling supply of volunteers, funding sources unable to match the demand and competition for scarce prevention resources. Nationwide, local, state and federal censorship of educational campaigns is a problem. In addition, various population groups are struggling for self-determination in the creation of culturally relevant prevention strategies. As the "face" of AIDS changes and includes more women, children, minorities and drug users, the problems will become even more complex. Communities still relatively untouched have the opportunity to begin this cooperative and collaborative approach before it is too late. Recent statistics clearly demonstrate that the epidemic is moving out of major cities and into smaller towns nationwide. Time is critical. The process will be a long and challenging one. But, community by community, we can bring an end to this devastating epidemic.

MERVYN F. SILVERMAN, MD, MPH
PRESIDENT, AMERICAN FOUNDATION FOR AIDS RESEARCH
DIRECTOR, THE ROBERT WOOD JOHNSON FOUNDATION
AIDS HEALTH SERVICES PROGRAM

Acknowledgments

We are indebted to a great many individuals and institutions for their contributions to *Ending the HIV Epidemic*.

From the very outset of the project, individuals on the frontlines in the fight to end the HIV epidemic were asked to take valuable time away from their work to help share with others the lessons of our fight in San Francisco. We could not have asked for a greater commitment of either time or spirit.

For their contributions to the development of the ideas and concepts in this book, we are immeasurably grateful to Patrick Biernacki, Henrik Blum, Cherrie Boyer, Joseph Cantania, Pat Christen, Wayne Clark, Thomas J. Coates, Harvey Feldman, Chuck Frutchey, Mindy Thompson Fullilove, Paul M. Gibson, (W.) Paul Gibson, Joseph Guydish, Katherine Haynes, Ernesto Hinojos, Stephen B. Hulley, Susan Kegeles, Philip R. Lee, Edward S. Morales, Steve Morin, George Lemp, Lyn Paleo, Mary Pittman-Lindeman, Mervyn

F. Silverman and Florence Stroud.

For overseeing the drafting and development of individual chapters, very special thanks go to Jeffery W. Amory, Margaret Chesney, Renata Kiefer and Ron Stall. Their patience was matched only by their pursuit of excellence. We are also deeply appreciative of the significant contributions of Larry Bye and Elizabeth Stoller to this project.

We would also like to acknowledge the following institutions and organizations for their commitment to the development of *Ending the HIV Epidemic*: The Robert Wood Johnson Foundation; Center for AIDS Prevention Studies, University of California, San Francisco; Institute for Health Policy Studies, University of California, San Francisco; Communication Technologies; MidCity Consortium to Combat AIDS; San Francisco Department of Public Health; and the San Francisco AIDS Foundation.

The making of any book always requires top-notch support staff. We have been more than fortunate to have had the expertise and dedication of Francis Jue, and especially Michael S. Broder, who toiled into the night more often than he would ever care to remember. Special thanks are also due to Karen Watnick, George Martin, John Tighe and Gail Wiley, as well as to our editors at ETR Associates/Network Publications, Kay Clark and Mary Nelson, each of whom helped bring this project to fruition. Their early and continued support was crucial to the completion of the book.

Sam B. Puckett was the original editor of this book. Sam was a community activist and educator with long and deep roots in San Francisco's fight against AIDS. Sam died of AIDS in the fall of 1988. Many of those associated with this project, however, still frequently refer to this as "Sam's book." We are very fortunate for the time we had Sam in our midst.

Finally, we would like to acknowledge all the "unnamed" San Franciscans who have worked long and hard to prevent the spread of HIV in our communities. To these soldiers in the fight, our deepest debt lies as does our greatest hope for ending the HIV epidemic.

—S.P.
—P.F.
—T.R.W.

Introduction

The making of *Ending the HIV Epidemic: Community Strategies in Disease Prevention and Health Promotion* has been a long, challenging and ultimately rewarding process. In 1986, The Robert Wood Johnson Foundation awarded a grant to the Institute for Health Policy Studies of the University of California, San Francisco, to establish an AIDS Resource Program. The purpose of the program was to assist communities outside San Francisco in responding to the HIV epidemic and to support San Francisco's public and private agencies in providing information and assistance to other communities throughout the United States. The seed monies to support the development of this book were made available through the AIDS Resource Program to the San Francisco AIDS Foundation.

Our purpose with this book is to provide readers—public health leaders, community organizers, policymakers, community-based agency directors and health educators—with the most accurate information and expert thought on developing prevention strategies to reduce the spread of HIV in communities throughout this nation. It is a book about San Francisco's efforts to develop a community-wide HIV prevention strategy, not about our comprehensive, community-based system of care and support for people with HIV disease. We also have limited our discussion to primary prevention, the prevention of HIV infection.

This is not a scholarly book. It is not targeted to the research community. It is not meant to sit on library shelves. It is targeted to those individuals who will be designing and implementing HIV prevention strategies in their communities. It is meant to be understandable and useful to the widest possible audience. *Ending the HIV Epidemic* is a book for people to read, to think about, to discuss with others and *then to act upon.*

It is clear that the HIV epidemic now poses a threat to an increasing number of communities throughout the United States. Lessons learned in San Francisco and elsewhere indicate that new strategies in health promotion and disease prevention will be required to halt the spread of HIV infection. Specifically, HIV prevention necessitates the broad and active involvement of members of all populations within the community directly affected by the epidemic. It also requires the involvement of many in the community whose lives are not directly affected by the epidemic in the development of prevention strategies and interventions.

Ending the HIV Epidemic is constructed in three parts. Part I, Understanding the HIV Epidemic, provides the basic foundation for understanding the emergence and the epidemiology of the epidemic. Chapter 1 presents a history of the HIV epidemic and what is currently known about HIV infection. Included is a discussion of previous epidemics, focusing on the influenza and polio epidemics earlier in this century, as well as efforts to combat sexually transmitted bacterial diseases such as syphilis and gonorrhea. The authors also examine the clinical spectrum of HIV disease.

Chapter 2 distinguishes three different aspects of the epidemic, which include HIV infection, clinically manifest HIV disease and the socioeconomic and political consequences of HIV infection and AIDS. Other discussions include the distribution of AIDS and HIV infection, prospects for the future, public health implications, preventing the spread of HIV infection and psychosocial and sociocultural issues in prevention.

The third chapter presents an overview of health promotion efforts in the United States during this century. This chapter examines the evolutionary changes in health promotion and illness prevention, placing programs directed toward HIV risk reduction in an historical and theoretical context. The authors discuss lessons from behavioral medicine and health promotion as they outline five stages of health promotion efforts.

Part I is intended to provide readers with the necessary grounding to understand the many facets of the HIV epidemic. Readers already familiar with these areas are encouraged to move directly to Part II, The San Francisco Response.

The three chapters comprising Part II detail different aspects of the prevention effort in San Francisco. Chapter 4 examines the prevention and risk-reduction aspects of the "San Francisco model" from 1982 to 1989. The author highlights the three dimensions of the overall prevention effort adopted by the San Francisco Department of Public Health, which includes detailed discussions of audiences, approaches and messages. This chapter also depicts how the overall prevention effort was coordinated, highlighting the partnership between the Department of Public Health and San Francisco's AIDS-focused community-based organizations.

Chapter 5 continues the discussion of the partnership between the Department of Public Health and community-based organizations with roots in the communities and subcultures most heavily affected by the epidemic. Specifically, challenges to that partnership are highlighted, including: the bathhouse controversy, HIV antibody testing, outreach to ethnic communities, the impact of bureaucratic expansion and the problem of censorship of materials.

Chapter 6 outlines the principles of effective program design that have emerged from nearly a decade's experience in San Francisco. Four areas of program design are discussed: approaches and messages, building relationships with target audiences, changing public policy and the role of research and evaluation.

Part III, Preventing the Spread of HIV in Your Community, consists of two chapters that provide nuts and bolts expertise concerning the development, design and implementation of prevention programs. Chapter 7 examines the general response of communities to the epidemic, factors influencing community response, stages in community response, the role of community planning, different types of planning for different purposes and 12 basic steps in the planning and implementation process at the community level.

The final chapter, Chapter 8, is a powerful essay written by a longtime San Francisco activist, AIDS educator and policymaker. The "call to action" lays out five challenges for communities responding to the HIV epidemic in the 1990s. The challenges include: community organizing, risk taking, embracing conflict, building partnerships and building leadership for coalitions.

This book is the product of the efforts of more than 35 San Francisco leaders who work to prevent the further spread of HIV infection. For the first time, men and women from nearly all of the city's diverse communities and populations sat down together to create a book that speaks for all of us. Institutions and agencies represented in the process of developing the book include the San Francisco Department of Public Health, the Institute for Health Policy Studies and Center for AIDS Prevention Studies at the University of California, San Francisco, interested private sector groups such as Communication Technologies, and community-based organizations, including MidCity Consortium to Combat AIDS and the San Francisco AIDS Foundation.

Our diversity of backgrounds, approaches and perspectives is not camouflaged in the following pages. We do not speak in a single voice, although there is much resonance in what we say. Over the last years, we have sat at common tables, early in the morning and after hours, to debate and to argue, to listen and to learn. The process has been as remarkable as the product.

Above all else, we have endeavored to make this book useful for people who want to act—to take the necessary steps to plan, to design, to implement and to evaluate HIV prevention programs in communities throughout the United States.

STEVEN PETROW
SAN FRANCISCO AIDS FOUNDATION

Part I
Understanding the HIV Epidemic

A Modern Epidemic Emerges: History and Context

Renata G. Kiefer and Stephen B. Hulley

INTRODUCTION

Acquired immunodeficiency syndrome (AIDS) is the end stage of the chronic infectious disease caused by the human immunodeficiency virus (HIV), a new and lethal retrovirus. AIDS has spread rapidly since being recognized in 1981. In the United States, the total number of AIDS cases reported to the Centers for Disease Control (CDC) was almost 118,000 by December 31, 1989. Ten times as many people may be infected with the virus who have not yet progressed to full-fledged disease.[1] More than 50 percent of all persons diagnosed with AIDS have died, more than 70,000 through December 1989.[2]

As of December 1989, the total number of AIDS cases reported to the World Health Organization (WHO) from 153 countries was 198,165—an underestimate, due to delays in reporting as well as common underreporting and underdiagnosis in many countries. Table 1 shows the distribution of AIDS cases in the world, with the majority in the Americas, primarily the United States. WHO estimates the true number of current AIDS cases to be approximately 600,000 worldwide, with six to eight million people infected with HIV.[3] The HIV epidemic poses an unprecedented threat to public health in any country, not only because of the large number of young lives that it claims and the burdens of illness and suffering it imposes on society, but also because it accentuates society's economic and sociopolitical ills, such as resource shortages and social strife.

The future dimensions of the epidemic depend a great deal on the measures society takes today. In the nine years since the description of the first AIDS cases, much has been learned through epidemiologic, biomedical and behavioral research. Although there is still no cure for AIDS and no vaccine to prevent its acquisition, transmission of the infection is known to occur only in very specific, limited ways through behaviors that can be modified. The major task at hand is to facilitate and bring about the behavioral changes necessary for prevention.

These first two chapters set forth what everyone—health care professionals, public policymakers, school district leaders or any other community leaders—should know about the nature of the disease, its modes of transmission and the evolving pattern of the epidemic in the United States, in order to develop sound preventive strategies for themselves, for their families and friends and for their communities.

AIDS: A NEW DISORDER

In the spring of 1981, the CDC received reports of *Pneumocystis carinii* pneumonia (PCP) and Kaposi's sarcoma (KS) occurring in two clusters of previously healthy young homosexual men in California and New York.[4] PCP is a rare infectious disease that occurs only in individuals with a depressed immune system (an opportunistic infection). KS is a rare cancer that previously occurred only in elderly men or in patients receiving immunosuppressive drugs. None

Table 1. DISTRIBUTION OF REPORTED CASES OF AIDS IN THE WORLD, BY COUNTRY

	N	Percent
Americas	**131,250**	**66%**
U.S.	110,333	
Brazil	7,787	
Canada	2,996	
Mexico	2,683	
Haiti	2,215	
All others	5,236	
Europe	**28,367**	**14%**
France	8,025	
Italy	4,663	
FR Germany	4,093	
Spain	3,965	
United Kingdom	2,649	
Switzerland	1,046	
Netherlands	983	
All others	2,943	
Africa	**36,279**	**18%**
Uganda	7,375	
Kenya	6,004	
Zaire	4,636	
Tanzania	4,158	
Malawi	2,586	
Burundi	1,975	
Zambia	1,892	
Rwanda	1,302	
All others	6,351	
Western Pacific	**1,902**	**1%**
East Mediterranean	**299**	**<<1%**
Southeast Asia	**68**	**<<1%**
Total	**198,165**	**100%**

Reported to WHO through December 1, 1989 (AIDS 1990; 4:93-97)

of these young patients had an underlying condition or had received drugs that could explain their immune depression.

By mid-1981 a special task force on opportunistic infections and Kaposi's sarcoma was created by the CDC to determine whether these conditions indicated a new disease and to set up surveillance. Intensive investigative efforts revealed a few additional cases of KS or PCP occurring in young people between 1978 and 1981 and a remarkable increase in the number of such patients starting in 1981. By 1982 Kaposi's sarcoma and/or an opportunistic infection in a person with unexplained immunodeficiency was determined to be a new disorder, subsequently called acquired immunodeficiency syndrome (AIDS).

Scientists asked: What factor or combination of factors could weaken the immune system of otherwise healthy men to such an extent as to make them subject to life-threatening opportunistic infections and a rare cancer? Searching for clues, case-control studies compared homosexual men who had AIDS with healthy homosexual men matched for age, race and geographic location.[5] The results suggested that men who had numerous sexual partners, frequented bathhouses or used intravenous drugs were at risk for AIDS.

In the meantime, AIDS had begun to appear in other population groups. The syndrome was reported in intravenous drug users in the latter part of 1981. Haitian immigrants with AIDS were reported in 1982; these were men and women who did not report being intravenous drug users or homosexuals. AIDS also began to appear in hemophiliacs, with cases reported from different parts of the United States, Canada and Europe; their only common element was the frequent need for transfusions of coagulation factor VIII, made from pooled blood donations.[6] AIDS was also reported in patients who had received a blood transfusion months to years prior to becoming ill; at least one high-risk donor was found in each case investigated.[7] Finally, AIDS began to appear in female partners of bisexual men or of intravenous drug users, and in their infants.

Of the first one thousand AIDS cases reported by February 1983, 72 percent were homosexual or bisexual men, 15 percent intravenous drug users, 5 percent were Haitian, 1 percent were hemophiliac and 6 percent were in none of these four groups.[8] Thus, while homosexual men accounted for the majority of persons with AIDS, this disease was not confined to the homosexual population. Scientists had previously postulated that repeated exposures to numerous infectious agents might so overload the immune system as to cause its eventual failure. The appearance of AIDS in recipients of blood transfusions favored the hypothesis of a new viral agent.

PATTERNS OF RISK:
PROTECTING THE BLOOD SUPPLY

On the basis of these occurrence patterns and in an effort to protect the blood supply and to stop the spread of the disease via contaminated blood, four population groups at risk were identified by the CDC in March 1983: homosexuals and bisexuals with multiple partners, intravenous drug users, recent Haitian immigrants and hemophiliacs. Other individuals considered at risk were the sexual partners of persons at risk for AIDS. Given that the causative agent of AIDS was not known and there was no laboratory test to determine who had the disease, members of these risk groups were asked to refrain from donating blood. Another recommendation was that sexual contact should be avoided "with persons known or suspected to have AIDS."[9]

Although the risk group designation for the purpose of voluntary blood donor deferral made sense, given the urgent need to protect the blood supply, there were unfortunate social implications for members of these four groups. Little was known at the time about the disease and what put people at risk, so that there was no way to differentiate members within each group. Thus, belonging to a high-risk group appeared tantamount to being at increased risk not only of acquiring the disease but also of having the disease and infecting others.[10] The association of a life-threatening disease with population groups often held in low esteem had the potential for increasing discrimination against these groups. The potential political and social consequences of the risk group label in this case were compounded by the erroneous notion that the transmission pattern of the postulated AIDS virus was very similar to that of hepatitis B, i.e., that it was transmitted not only through blood or sexual intercourse but also through close household contact.[11]

ISOLATING THE VIRUS

In the spring of 1983, two years after the first AIDS cases had been described, the viral agent was isolated for the first time from a swollen lymph node of a patient. Intensive research over the following 19 months established that this virus was the cause and not the consequence of AIDS.[12] Once laboratories were able to grow the virus in cell cultures in sufficient quantities for research purposes,[13] antibody screening tests could be developed. Serologic screening of blood donors was instituted in March 1985.

Serologic testing permitted the diagnosis of HIV infection in asymptomatic individuals and over time revealed the wide spectrum of HIV disease, including a prolonged asymptomatic phase of many years. Moreover, further research showed that while hepatitis B can be transmitted in close household contact, this is not the case for HIV. Epidemiologic studies have shown that HIV can be transmitted through blood, sexual intercourse and from mother to newborn, but that HIV is not transmitted through touching, sneezing or other forms of contact. (See Chapter 2 for full discussion of how the virus is transmitted.)

But early images have been difficult to change, and the notion of contagion through casual contact continues to linger. Children with AIDS are often still seen as "contaminators" of schools, and adult members of risk groups as potential dangers at the work place. Much work remains to be done to correct misconceptions about this disease and to build safeguards against actions based on ignorance or prejudice, so that effective preventive efforts can be implemented.

Although there is still no cure for AIDS, inroads have been made in the treatment of opportunistic infections and in antiviral therapy that may slow the progression of disease in infected individuals. Biomedical approaches to prevention of infection have been less successful, and preventive efforts in the foreseeable future will not have the help of a vaccine. However, the modes of HIV transmission depend on human behavior, and further spread of the epidemic is preventable to the extent that approaches to changing behaviors and group norms in the community are successful.

THE HIV EPIDEMIC IN CONTEXT

By definition, an epidemic is an increase in the frequency of a disease occurring in a population in excess of what would normally be expected. Every epidemic must be seen in the particular social context in which it took hold, in order to understand both its propagation and society's response to it.

The propagation of an infectious disease epidemic in a population depends on the number of contagious individuals (those who are capable of transmitting the infection) and susceptible individuals (those who are capable of becoming infected), on the modes of transmission of the infection and on the infectious dose required for transmission. Propagation also depends on prevailing customs—individual and collective behaviors—that may create favorable opportunities for transmission.[14]

Historically, epidemics abate when the number of contagious individuals declines due to death or effective treatment or when the number of susceptible individuals falls due to the development of natural immunity or by vaccination. Epidemics may also abate as a result of changes in the ecologic conditions, including customs and behaviors, that initially favored propagation. While identification of the infectious agent is essential for the development of vaccines and biomedical treatment, all that is needed for effective public health intervention is to know the mode of transmission.

The HIV epidemic will not abate due to a decline in the number of contagious individuals in the next few years, because of the prolonged silent incubation period (currently known to last many years) and the absence of a cure. The epidemic cannot abate by a loss of susceptible individuals because the disease does not appear to cause a state of immunity (this is one of the reasons for pessimism about the prospects for an effective vaccine). However, given our knowledge of the modes of transmission, the epidemic can be prevented in the long run by community-wide changes in those customs and behaviors that facilitate the spread of HIV infection.

Epidemics: A Phenomenon of the Past?

It is instructive to review the history of how society has managed prior epidemics. Plagues have periodically swept across countries throughout history, but such events had become less common by the twentieth century. General improvements in living conditions, such as less crowding, improved sanitation and better nutrition, created a less favorable environment for plagues. These improvements were responsible for much of the declining mortality from diseases such as tuberculosis, cholera and diphtheria,[15] even prior to the development of drugs and vaccines to combat infectious diseases. Finally, the antibiotic era beginning around World War II raised hopes that every infectious disease would eventually be treatable or preventable by a pharmacologic magic bullet.

Thus, by the early 1980s, widespread infectious disease epidemics were thought to be a phenomenon of the past in developed countries, due not only to the improved standards of living but also to the extraordinary biomedical and technological advances of the past 40 years. The wide range of potent antimicrobial drugs to treat infectious diseases and effective vaccines to prevent many of them created the expectation that existing research capacities would be able to rise to any new challenge. Moreover, an epidemic surveillance network linked public health agencies throughout the country with the federal Centers for Disease Control, which leads the world in its early detection and prompt investigation of any disease outbreak and in its swift remedial action. In general, infectious diseases were perceived as having specific causes that could be found and eradicated.

A good example to illustrate the evolution of this view is polio, a disease caused by a virus that (like other viruses, including HIV) is not sensitive to the antibiotics that have been so successful in treating bacterial diseases. However, the development of effective and safe vaccines in the 1950s has led to the virtual eradication of this disease in populations of developed countries. Another example is influenza, which killed approximately 600,000 people in the United States and an estimated 20 million worldwide during the influenza pandemic of 1918-19.[16] Since influenza is an acute respiratory viral infection readily transmitted by respiratory droplet spread, this epidemic may have been favored by concentrations of people in close quarters during the war effort. Improved standards of living, the capacity to treat bacterial complications and the availability of vaccines make another epidemic of such magnitude unlikely today.

Syphilis and Gonorrhea

An example of particular relevance to the HIV epidemic in terms of social reactions is the epidemic of sexually transmitted bacterial diseases, syphilis and gonorrhea. Both diseases have been known for centuries, and until the introduction of penicillin in the 1940s, there was no effective treatment for either. Two important lessons can be learned from the example of these diseases: First, attempts to enforce moral codes by the threat of disease will not prevent the spread of diseases that depend on individual behaviors, nor will compulsory measures, such as quarantines, control an epidemic of such diseases. Second, the availability of an effective treatment alone cannot prevent further spread of such diseases.

At the beginning of World War I, 13 percent of United States draftees were reported to have either syphilis or gonorrhea.[17] The most important obstacle to halting the spread of these diseases was not the lack of an effective drug but the conspiracy of silence imposed by Victorian moral concepts, which forced people with venereal diseases underground and led to misconceptions about the diseases and their mode of spread. Explicit education was not allowed for fear of offending societal proprieties. Notions abounded that syphilis could be spread casually by pens, pencils, toilet seats, drinking cups and doorknobs (the U.S. Navy even removed doorknobs from its battle ships during World War I).[18]

Venereal disease, at the time, was considered just punishment for unwholesome ways of life and low moral standards.[19] Condoms were not made available for prophylaxis, because they were believed to promote increased sexual activity. Instead, the military established sanitary stations for urethral injections of disinfectant after presumed exposure, a painful and punitive procedure. More than 20,000 prostitutes were quarantined to segregate them from potential customers, and venereal disease in a soldier was an offense subject to court-martial.[20] In spite of these Draconian measures, the rates of disease did not abate.

Controlling Venereal Disease

In the 1930s, progress was made in the control of syphilis, under the leadership of Surgeon General Thomas Parran, with a program designed to find cases, treat them and educate the public. Centers providing free, confidential syphilis serology testing were expanded, and new facilities were established to serve those who could not afford to pay for their treatment. There was a reduction of the death rate from syphilis, from 19 per 100,000 population in 1918 to 16 per 100,000 in 1938.[21] Moreover, concerns about fitness of soldiers during World War II stimulated more enlightened educational programs, condom distribution and non-punitive treatment.[22]

After penicillin became available in 1943, the incidence of both syphilis and gonorrhea began to fall, reaching very low levels by the end of the 1950s; syphilis fell to 4 cases per 100,000 population by 1956.[23] Expectations that the "single-shot cure" would eradicate these diseases altogether led to a reduction of public funding and dismantling of existing disease control structures.[24] Increasing rates of syphilis during the 1960s reflected the increased sexual activity of the population (the "sexual revolution"), and there has been a sharp increase since 1985, which has been associated with a growing problem with crack cocaine and other recreational drugs.[25] In 1985 there were 28 civilian cases of syphilis per 100,000 U.S. population; but by 1988 the number of cases had increased to 42 civilian cases per 100,000 U.S. population.[26] These statistics show that the availability of a curative treatment alone is insufficient for the control of diseases that are behaviorally mediated.[27] They also illustrate both the importance of and the difficulty in developing an effective population-wide approach to behavior change.

As a result of the full spectrum of public health advances, however, the proportion of overall mortality attributable to infectious disease has become very small relative to chronic diseases in most developed countries. Thus, whereas in 1900 infectious diseases accounted for more than one-third of all deaths in developed countries, by 1970 this figure had shrunk to 2 percent, with cardiovascular diseases accounting for 45 percent and cancer for 18 percent.[28] Smoking and diet are now recognized as major determinants of these prevalent noninfectious diseases, and recent public health efforts have focused on studying these behaviors and how best to modify them.[29] This growing awareness of the importance of behavior change techniques has created an appropriate background for creating effective strategies to prevent the further spread of HIV infection.

HIV: THE NATURAL HISTORY

The Virus

HIV is a new human retrovirus. Its origin is unknown and shrouded in mystery, although it has been subject to much speculation.[30] Two viral subtypes are currently known: HIV-1, the original and most common subtype, and HIV-2, recovered in 1985 from West African patients with AIDS and more recently in Europe and North America from persons who have lived in West Africa.[31] Many of the complex molecular and biological features of HIV-1 have been characterized in recent years. Less is currently known about HIV-2, but it appears to be transmitted by the same modes and to require the same preventive measures. The term HIV in the subsequent discussion refers to HIV-1.

HIV has the capacity of infecting and reproducing in several human cell types, particularly in cells of the immune defense system and cells of the central nervous system. The virus preferentially infects cells carrying the CD4 molecule, which serves as a receptor facilitating viral entry into the cell. CD4 appears to be present on the surface of many cells, in particular first-line immune defense cells such as T-helper lymphocytes and macrophages, and possibly also interstitial support cells found in the central nervous system. Several unique molecular and biologic features such as latency, heterogeneity, direct cell-to-cell transmission and capacity for immune suppression contribute to the variable pattern of disease progression once infection has occurred. They may also play a role in transmission of the infection.

Once inside a living cell, the retroviral properties of HIV allow it to reproduce by transforming its own genetic material in such a way that it integrates into the genetic code of the cell. Infection of the host cell appears to be permanent, and whenever the cell divides, the viral code is passed on to each of the daughter cells. The virus may remain dormant in this form for a long time, or it may induce the cellular machinery to produce multiple copies of new virus that are released to infect other cells. The capacity of the viral genetic material to remain dormant in the host cell explains the long latency period between infection and the development of clinically manifest disease.[32] Recent studies have shown that there appears to be no period when HIV is dormant in all infected cells.[33] Thus, individuals are potentially capable of transmitting the infection even if they have no symptoms. Moreover, cells harboring latent virus may persist as circulating reservoirs of HIV capable of transmitting the infection to another person.[34]

Heterogeneity reflects the capacity of HIV to change over time, which is thought to be due to a high rate of mutation during viral replication.[35] Numerous strains have been isolated, even from the same individual at the same time and at different times.[36] Strains may differ in the protein structure of their envelope and thereby escape detection by the immune defense system. They may differ in infectivity (the ability to penetrate different target cells), in virulence (the ability to replicate in cells and cause damage) or in latency (the ability to remain dormant in infected cells).[37] Host-virus interactions are determinants of when, where and how HIV infection will progress to clinical disease in an individual and probably influence the transmissibility of the infection to other individuals. HIV strains isolated from patients over time have shown changes in virulence, ranging from a waxing and waning capacity to replicate in cell cultures to an increase in viral damage-causing properties demonstrated in isolates obtained at a later stage of disease.[38]

Infected cells can fuse with other cells and transfer HIV directly to another cell. Since the virus does not have to enter the extracellular space in this process, it is not exposed to antibodies.[39] During sexual intercourse, the virus may be transmitted by fusion of infected cells with cells present in an open lesion of the uninfected partner, particularly if inflammation is present in the lesion. These biologic and molecular features render the development of an effective vaccine against HIV extremely difficult and may also limit the usefulness of drugs, because of the potential emergence of resistant mutants.

Most of the disease-producing capacity of HIV is due to its propensity to infect and destroy cells essential for immune regulation and appropriate immune defense, notably T-helper (T4) lymphocytes. Destruction of immune cells occurs progressively over time, most likely through repeated bursts of viral multiplication; the mechanisms turning such viral proliferation on and off are not well understood.[40] When an infected cell is stimulated into an active state, virus can replicate into multiple copies, destroy the cell and spread to infect other target cells.

One theory is that any challenge to the immune defense system, either from another infectious agent or from reinfection with HIV, may activate cells harboring latent HIV. It appears that HIV can interfere with the normal function of healthy cells, as well as mislead the body's immune defense into destroying uninfected T4 cells.[41] The progressive loss of immune function culminates in a profound and permanent immunodeficiency, thus favoring the development of Kaposi's sarcoma and other malignant tumors and *pneumocystis* pneumonia and other opportunistic infections with organisms that would not usually cause disease in a person with an uncompromised immune system.

Antibodies to HIV usually develop within three months of infection (seroconversion), but occasionally it may take six months or even longer for antibodies to be demonstrated in the blood. Most knowledge of the time to seroconversion has been derived from transfusion recipients who had received contaminated blood, since the time of infection could be determined in these cases. The time of HIV infection acquired by other means is usually much more difficult to pinpoint. The occurrence of infected persons in whom antiviral antibodies do not develop in the first three to six months after infection is not well established and probably rare.[42] The time between acquisition of the virus and seroconversion is a window during which HIV infection cannot be diagnosed by antibody testing.

Antibodies to HIV are not protective. In contrast to most other infectious diseases caused by viral agents, for which antibodies indicate a protective immune response and clearing of the virus from the bloodstream, HIV persists in the bloodstream in spite of the presence of antibodies.[43]

There are currently several types of serologic assays for the detection of antibodies to HIV. The most widely used serologic testing procedure for laboratory diagnosis of HIV infection is the enzyme-linked immunosorbent assay (ELISA), combined with a confirmatory test such as the Western blot. Other tests are being developed to detect the presence of virus or of viral components in body fluids, rather than detecting antibodies to the virus. These tests are used in specialized centers for specific research purposes and are not suitable for screening purposes at this time.[44]*

For initial screening, the ELISA is used. Under good laboratory conditions, the ELISA has a high sensitivity, more than 99 percent (i.e., the test is positive for HIV antibodies in almost all sera of infected individuals who have developed antibodies). Thus, the rate of false negatives will be extremely low. In population groups with high prevalence of HIV infection, a positive ELISA is highly predictive of HIV infection. This is less true for populations with a low prevalence, where many positive results will turn out to be false positives.

In order to improve the specificity of HIV testing, i.e., to reduce the false positive rate, the following testing sequence has been established. Serum samples are first tested for HIV antibodies by ELISA, and if the result is positive, the ELISA is repeated. If the repeat is also positive, a Western blot test is performed for confirmation. If the ELISA is positive but the Western blot is indeterminate or negative, testing is repeated at a later date, in order to avoid false negatives.[47]

A positive result after this sequence has an extremely high predictive value for HIV infection, even in low prevalence general populations,[48] provided that the confirmatory testing is carried out in a

---

* Procedures to detect virus or viral components have been applied to test body fluids from infected individuals' blood, serum, semen, vaginal/cervical secretions, cerebrospinal fluid, breast milk, urine, saliva, tears, lung fluid and amniotic fluid. Virus has been isolated from all types of fluid tested, but in very different concentrations. Cerebrospinal fluid, blood and semen had the highest concentrations, whereas only minute quantities of virus were found in tears, saliva and urine.[45] Only blood, semen, vaginal/cervical secretions and breast milk have been implicated in transmission of the infection.[46] Virus-infected cells may be the major vehicle of HIV transmission in genital fluid.[46] These biologic findings corroborate the epidemiologic evidence that HIV infection is transmitted only through contact with blood, through intimate sexual contact or from an infected mother to her newborn infant through perinatal events.

high-quality reference laboratory with experienced personnel. This high specificity is important for establishing an individual diagnosis, in order to avoid the tragic implications of a false positive result.

The Clinical Spectrum

For surveillance purposes, AIDS is defined by the CDC as the presence of a reliably diagnosed disease indicative of an underlying deficiency in the immune system in the absence of an illness or drugs known to cause immunosuppression. The initial case definition of 1982 was narrower, requiring biopsy-proven KS or biopsy/culture-proven PCP. The subsequent development of laboratory methods to detect HIV led to an increasing awareness of the broad spectrum of HIV-related disease. In 1985 and again in 1987, the CDC surveillance case definition was expanded to include certain other illnesses if they occur in an HIV seropositive individual, such as other opportunistic infections, cancers of the lymphoid tissue, brain disorders, a wasting syndrome, and in children under 13 years of age, recurrent severe bacterial diseases.[49]

In the United States, cases of AIDS are reported to local and state health departments and then to CDC. This reporting system gives a reasonably complete count, although considerable underreporting has been documented in some regions and some populations.[50] Moreover, HIV-related illnesses that do not meet the CDC AIDS case definition, such as bacterial pneumonias in injection drug users,[51] account for a significant proportion of HIV-related morbidity and mortality. Thus, reported AIDS cases likely represent less than 80 percent of all HIV-associated morbidity,[52] and this proportion appears to be lower in ethnic populations.[53]

The spectrum of HIV disease ranges from infection without any symptoms to the clinical manifestations of AIDS, and the clinical course may vary considerably from one individual to another. A substantial proportion of infected persons develop nonspecific symptoms of an acute flu-like illness within a few weeks after becoming infected. Many infected individuals then remain asymptomatic for many years (latency period), while a few progress to severe end-stage disease within two years.[54]

Why such differences exist is unknown. It is also not known what proportion of infected individuals remain asymptomatic for a long time, since such persons are often unaware of their infection unless they perceive themselves at risk and seek antibody testing. Some infected persons come to medical attention because of chronic symptoms, such as persistent swelling of lymph nodes, but many present initially with an opportunistic infection or an AIDS-associated cancer.

Data from homosexual populations indicate that about 50 percent of infected adults develop clinical AIDS within ten years; current estimates of the median latency period for AIDS are between eight and eleven years.[55] It is not known what proportion of the remaining 50 percent of infected adults will develop AIDS or whether some infected individuals will never do so. The length of the latency period is considerably longer than estimates based on observations made earlier in the epidemic, when those with longer incubation periods had not yet become ill.[56] Treatment with the antiviral drug zidovudine (AZT) has been shown to slow disease progression and may prolong the latency period in the future.[57]

Initial disease manifestation is important for prognosis in adults; patients presenting with Kaposi's sarcoma have had a longer median survival duration than those with PCP. Median survival following the diagnosis of PCP has been estimated to be between nine and thirteen months, with a terminal wasting illness involving fever, adenopathy, diarrhea and weight loss; survival beyond four years may be less than 5 percent. Survival has also been shown to vary with gender, age, ethnic group, risk group and response to treatment of opportunistic infections and to antiviral therapy.[58] Median survival has shown increases for adult patients diagnosed since 1986, particularly those with PCP,[59] probably due to effective new therapies such as AZT to slow progression of HIV disease and aerosolized pentamidine to prevent and treat PCP.

Prognosis in children varies both with the age at which infection was acquired and the age at which symptoms occur. Survival is longer in children infected after two years of age than for those infected earlier in life or prior to birth.[60] The median age of clinical onset of disease in perinatally infected infants is eight months; mortality is highest in the first year of life; and median survival time after diagnosis was 38 months in one recent study.[61]

With mounting evidence that AZT slows disease progression in both symptomatic and asymptomatic infected persons and with recent improvements in the treatment and prophylaxis against opportunistic infections, early diagnosis and therapy become increasingly important in efforts to reduce morbidity in both children and adults with HIV infection.

2

Patterns of the Epidemic and Public Health Implications

Renata G. Kiefer, Joseph R. Guydish,
Katherine C. Haynes, George F. Lemp
and Stephen B. Hulley

INTRODUCTION

Three aspects of the epidemic can be distinguished.[1] The first is HIV infection (without symptoms), which had its onset in the mid-1970s. Its future rate of growth is difficult to predict, but it will depend on the success of primary prevention through behavior modification. The second is clinically manifest HIV disease (with symptoms) with onset in the early 1980s. Its growth will continue in the next decade, even if no further spread of HIV infection were to occur, as the large pool of asymptomatic infected individuals (estimated to be ten times the number who have developed AIDS) becomes clinically ill.

The third aspect of the epidemic consists of the socioeconomic and political consequences of HIV infection and AIDS, with onset in the mid-1980s and as yet unpredictable but probably large future ramifications. The future extent of this third aspect of the epidemic will depend on the course of the other two. However, it will also depend on society's ability to overcome social strife, to provide leadership and funding and to bridle prejudicial and coercive tendencies in favor of mobilizing cooperative efforts, so an effective preventive response can be mounted to halt the further spread of the infection and to care for people with HIV disease.

In this chapter, the characteristics of these aspects of the epidemic in the United States will be discussed. Prevention strategies can be more effective if they are based on an understanding of the distribution patterns—the where, when and who of the disease outbreaks.

DISTRIBUTION OF AIDS

The number of AIDS cases in the United States has increased steadily over the past nine years, although the rate of increase has

Table 1. DISTRIBUTION OF REPORTED AIDS CASES
in the United States, by Standard Metropolitan Statistical Area of Residence, 1981-1989

	AIDS Cases		Adult population (millions)	Rate per 1000
	N	%		
New York, NY	22,665	19.2%	9.1	2.5
San Francisco, CA	7,386	6.3%	3.2	2.3
Los Angeles, CA	8,256	7%	7.5	1.1
Houston, TX	3,432	2.9%	2.9	1.2
Newark, NJ	3,354	2.9%	2.0	1.7
Washington, DC	3,303	2.8%	3.0	1.1
Chicago, IL	2,916	2.4%	7.1	.4
Miami, FL	2,995	2.5%	1.6	1.9
All others	63,474	54%	132.2	.5
Total	**117,781**	**100%**	**168.6**	**.7**

Reported to CDC through December 31, 1989.
CDC. HIV/AIDS Surveillance, January 1990.

declined gradually. The geographic distribution of AIDS still shows the largest number of cases in the urban epicenters that were the first to be affected; eight metropolitan areas account for almost one-half of all cases (Table 1). About one-fourth of the cases have occurred in New York and Newark, N.J., which together report almost twice the number of cases of San Francisco and Los Angeles combined. However, the geographic distribution of AIDS has shifted over time, reflecting the spread of the epidemic out of the epicenters. In 1984 New York, California, Florida, New Jersey, Texas and Illinois accounted for more than 80 percent all AIDS cases, but by the end of 1989 these states accounted for less than 60 percent.[2] Every state has reported AIDS cases, and 86 percent of the states have at least one hundred cases.[3]

The age distribution of AIDS has remained stable over time, reflecting the modes of transmission. Most AIDS patients are young, nearly one-half are between 30-39 years of age, one-fifth are in the 20-29 age group, another fifth are 40-49 years old, one-tenth are older than 50 and one-fiftieth are younger than 20 years of age.[4]

The sex distribution of AIDS in the United States and Western Europe reflects the initial modes of spread, i.e., among homosexual men and populations using injection drugs. Thus, the male to female ratio exceeds ten to one in the United States. The male preponderance exists also among adolescent AIDS cases, but in a ratio of only five to one.[5] The proportion of adult female AIDS cases has been increasing steadily from 8 percent of reported cases in 1987 to 10 percent in 1988 and 11 percent in 1989.[6]

The distribution of AIDS by risk group is strongly influenced by gender (Table 2). Among men, homosexual and bisexual men comprised 67 percent of AIDS cases in 1989; injection drug users constituted another 18 percent; and those who are both homosexual and injection drug users comprised 8 percent. Only 2 percent of men acquired their infection via heterosexual contact. Among women, on the other hand, more than half acquired their disease via injection drug use and a large proportion, 31 percent, contracted HIV infection as a result of heterosexual contact with an infected man.

The racial distribution of AIDS reveals that Black and Hispanic populations are disproportionately affected by this disease. Twenty-

Table 2. DISTRIBUTION OF REPORTED AIDS CASES
by Exposure Categories in the United States, 1981-1989

Risk group	% of AIDS cases			
	Men (N=105,175)	Women (N=10,611)	Children <13 yrs (N=1,995)	Total (N=117,781)
Homosexual contact with HIV	67%			61%
IV drug users (IVDU)	18%	52%		21%
Homosexual and IVDU	8%			7%
Transfusion recipient	2%	10%	11%	2%
Heterosexual contact with HIV	2%	31%		5%
Mother with HIV			81%	1%
Hemophiliac	1%		5%	1%
Undetermined	3%	7%	3%	3%
Total	100%	100%	100%	100%

CDC. HIV/AIDS Surveillance, January 1990.

seven percent of all AIDS patients are Black, whereas Blacks comprise only about 12 percent of the United States population. Similarly, although Hispanics comprise only 8 percent of the United States population, they represent 15 percent of all persons with AIDS.[7] The disproportionate involvement of ethnic populations is particularly severe for women and children; almost three-fourths of women with AIDS are Black or Hispanic, and nearly three-fourths of children with AIDS are Black or Hispanic (Table 3). Moreover, ethnic minorities are also disproportionately affected within each risk group, particularly among injection drug users with AIDS and among those who acquired AIDS by heterosexual contact.[8]

The majority of persons with AIDS are young adults in the prime of their productive years. Although children and adolescents with AIDS comprise only a small proportion of the total, the occurrence of AIDS in these young age groups has important public health implications. Children currently account for only 2 percent of all AIDS cases, but their number is growing, due to increasing numbers of infections transmitted from infected mothers to their newborns.[9]

Table 3. DISTRIBUTION OF REPORTED AIDS CASES
in the United States by Race and Sex, 1981-1989

Race	% of AIDS cases			U.S. Population	
	Men (N = 105,175)	Women (N = 10,611)	Children <13 yrs (N = 1,995)	≥15 yrs	<15 yrs
White	60%	27%	22%	81%	73%
Black	25%	52%	53%	11%	15%
Latino	15%	20%	25%	6%	9%
Other	1%	<1%	<1%	2%	3%
Total	100%	100%	100%	100%	100%

CDC. MMWR 1989; 38(S-4)
CDC. HIV/AIDS Surveillance Report, January 1990.

With perinatal transmission rates of HIV infection of 20 to 50 percent, this implies a two- to five-fold higher rate of maternal infections. Recent anonymous newborn screening data show wide regional differences, even in cities with high-risk populations. In New York City, 1 in 77 live births occurred to a seropositive mother, whereas in San Francisco it was 1 in 776 live births.[10]

Adolescents from 13 to 19 years of age comprise an even smaller proportion of AIDS patients, 0.4 percent in December 1988, but adolescents are a particularly vulnerable segment of society. With incubation periods of ten years or longer, the much higher proportion of persons with AIDS in the 20- to 24-years age group (4 percent) reflects infection acquired during adolescence.[11] Moreover, increasing crack cocaine use among segments of the adolescent population is an ominous sign for the future development of HIV infection in this population.[12]

A recent study of adolescents with AIDS[13] showed the mode of acquisition of HIV to vary with age and race as follows: Blood and blood products were the source of HIV for more than one-half of cases in 13 to 14 year olds, but for only one-fifth of the 17- to 19-years age group. Sexual contact or injection drug use accounted for one-tenth of cases among 13 to 14 year olds and more than one-half in the 17- to 19-years age group. Among adolescents the disproportionate involvement of ethnic groups is similar to that in adults, with Blacks and Hispanics comprising 34 percent and 17 percent of adolescent AIDS cases but only 14 percent and 8 percent of the United States population between 13 and 19 years of age.

DISTRIBUTION OF HIV INFECTION

The prevalence of HIV-infected persons in the United States, or indeed anywhere in the world, is not precisely known. Since AIDS has been a reportable disease in all 50 states, prevalence estimates for AIDS have been based on reported numbers, taking into account the probable degree of underreporting. Cases of HIV infection that do not meet the CDC case definition for AIDS have not been reportable in all states, so that individuals desiring antibody testing could do so with minimal risk of loss of confidentiality. Thus, information on the prevalence of people with HIV antibodies is based on various samples of the population, such as risk group estimates and several large population samples, each with its own sources of bias. Awareness of these biases is important in order to understand the meaning of the resulting estimates.[14]

Estimates Based on Studies of High-Risk Groups

The 1987 CDC estimate of 1-1.5 million infected persons in the United States was derived from estimates of the size and seroprevalence of the different risk groups: homosexual and bisexual men, intravenous drug users,* hemophiliacs, heterosexuals, and other groups such as transfusion recipients and partners of individuals at risk (Table 4). This corresponds to an infection rate of 0.4-0.6 percent (1 in 250 to 1 in 167 persons) in the total United States population of 245 million or 0.7-1.1 percent in the United States population between 17 and 54 years of age.[15] The estimate of HIV infection in the United States has recently been revised downward to between 700,000 and 1.31 million on the basis of an observed slowing in the rate of increase of reported AIDS cases in mid-1987, particularly in

---

* The CDC has always and continues to refer to "intravenous drug users" rather than the term "injection drug user."

homosexual and bisexual men who were not intravenous drug users.[16]

HIV seroprevalence remains highest in those groups that account for the majority of AIDS cases in the United States. A number of studies have addressed HIV infection in homosexual and bisexual

---

Table 4. CDC ESTIMATE OF NUMBER INFECTED WITH HIV
in the United States, 1987 (CDC, 1987)

Population	Estimated Size	Approximate Seroprevalence	N Infected
Homosexual (exclusively)	2,500,000	20-25%	500,000-625,000
Homosexual (occasional)	2,500,000-7,500,000	5%	125,000-375,000
IV drug use (regular)	900,000	25%	225,000
IV drug use (occasional)	200,000	5%	10,000
Hemophilia A	12,400	70%	8,700
Hemophilia B	3,100	35%	1,100
Heterosexuals (no known risk)	142,000,000	.021%	30,000
		Subtotal	900,000-1,270,000
Heterosexual contacts of above (5-10% of total infections)			45,000-127,000
		Total	945,000-1,400,000

---

men and in injection drug users. The seroprevalence rates in homosexual and bisexual men are generally between 20-50 percent.[17] The seroprevalence rates among all men living in cities like New York and San Francisco that have large numbers of high-risk residents may be as high as 10 percent, or 50 to 60 percent among homosexual men. High rates are reported in studies conducted in special settings such as STD clinics, and are likely to overestimate the true seroprevalence in the homosexual and bisexual population.[18] Studies over time have shown encouraging results. In San Francisco, seroconversion rates have decreased from 18 percent per year in 1982 to less than 1 percent per year in 1987, accompanied by a decrease in high-risk sexual practices.[19]

HIV seroprevalence among injection drug users is very high (50-60 percent) in the cities of the Northeast, particularly New York and Newark.[20] Infection rates in other parts of the country are lower than in the Northeast, generally 3 to 20 percent.[21] "Shooting galleries," where individuals meet to share and shoot drugs, may have led to high infection rates among injection drug users in the Northeast.[22] However, sharing of needles and syringes is common also among injection drug users in areas with as yet low seroprevalence.[23] Infected injection drug users have been a major link in the spread of the HIV epidemic into heterosexual populations,[24] and more than 70 percent of infants with AIDS have been born to mothers who were injection drug users (IDUs) or sexual partners of IDUs.[25]

Infection rates in heterosexual partners of infected persons are highly variable. Among persons who often have shared hundreds of episodes of unprotected vaginal intercourse, seroconversion rates have ranged from 0-58 percent, with a median of 24 percent. In a California partners study, 24 percent of 132 female partners of infected men and none of 20 male partners of infected women had antibody evidence of infection.[26] These findings illustrate the low infectivity of the virus through heterosexual intercourse in the United States—averaging about 1 in 500 episodes of unprotected vaginal intercourse between an infected and an uninfected person.[27] Infectivity appears to be higher with anal intercourse, and it is also much higher with vaginal intercourse when there are open sores on the genitalia.

Estimates Based on Surveys of Other Populations

Several surveys have addressed the issue of HIV prevalence in large population segments: blood donors, military recruits and child-bearing women. Seroprevalence among first-time blood donors is very low—less than 0.1 percent[28]—due to the voluntary self-deferral of individuals who are members of one of the high-risk groups listed in Table 2. It therefore underestimates the overall seroprevalence in the general population.

Since October 1985, the Department of Defense has screened all civilian applicants to military service for evidence of HIV. More than 1.7 million recruits (86 percent men) had been screened by

September 1988, with an overall seroprevalence of 0.14 percent. Men had a higher rate (0.15 percent) than women (0.07 percent). Black recruits were over five times and Hispanics over three times more likely to test positive than Whites.[29] Military screening probably underestimates seroprevalence in the general population. Homosexual and bisexual men and injection drug users are not eligible for military service and are underrepresented, while minorities and persons of lower socioeconomic status are over represented.

The geographic distribution of HIV infection in both military recruits and blood donors is similar to that of AIDS, with states reporting the highest rates of AIDS cases also having the higher seroprevalence in military recruits and blood donors.[30] The five-fold higher rates of HIV seroprevalence in men compared to women after adjusting for age and race is difficult to interpret, since the self-selection biases may be different for men and women.[31] Most of the seropositive individuals found among blood donors or military recruits have risk factors that fit into one of the described risk groups (Table 2). HIV infection in the United States among persons who do not know themselves to be in a high-risk group has been estimated to be low, 0.01-0.02 percent.[32]

The most representative large population surveys conducted in the United States are several statewide programs that test all women giving birth via anonymous testing of newborn blood samples. Since maternal HIV antibodies are transmitted to the fetus, their presence in newborn blood demonstrates that the mother is infected. HIV prevalence rates range from less than 0.1 percent in California, Colorado, Michigan, New Mexico and Texas to 0.2 percent in Massachusetts, 0.5 percent in Florida and New Jersey and 0.7 percent in New York. Since testing of infants is anonymous, there is no information about maternal risk factors. However, infection rates were highest among mothers delivering in metropolitan areas and lowest in rural areas.[33] Rates from 2-2.4 percent were reported from New York City zip codes known for high rates of drug use, and even higher rates were reported from several inner-city hospitals.[34]

These surveys of newborns also show much higher seroprevalence rates in Blacks and Hispanics than in Whites.[35] In one inner-city New York hospital, the rate in Black mothers was 5.6 times and in

Hispanic mothers 3.7 times the rate in White mothers.[36] This disproportionate involvement of ethnic minorities is also known to exist within risk groups.[37]

Information about HIV infection in adolescents is available from screening of all Job Corps applicants. The Job Corps provides residential training for disadvantaged youths between 14 and 21 years of age, but excludes active intravenous drug users. About 84,000 applicants have been tested since screening started in March 1987. Preliminary results released in May 1989 indicate an HIV seroprevalence rate of 0.41 percent.[38] Additional recent data cited from the CDC's national hospital survey indicate that as many as 1 percent of 15 to 16 year olds may be HIV-infected in high prevalence areas such as New York and Miami (patients admitted for trauma or substance abuse were not included in the study).[39]*

PROSPECTS FOR THE FUTURE

Any projection of the future course of the HIV epidemic will necessarily be based on imperfect knowledge and will at best yield a range of possibilities. Several methods have been used to forecast future numbers of affected individuals over the short term (two to five years).[42] Extrapolation uses current AIDS surveillance data and assumes that previous trends will continue to predict the cumulative number of AIDS cases in the future. Back calculation works backward from the number of observed AIDS cases and knowledge of the incubation period to estimate the number currently infected with HIV and predict the number of future AIDS cases. The reliability of any method decreases with efforts to predict the more distant future.

Based on estimates of the current number of HIV-infected individuals in the United States, the number of AIDS cases can be expected to increase tenfold in the 1990s even if no further spread of

---

* Substantial proportions of adolescents are sexually active and high-risk sexual behaviors are common.[40] Recent surveys of adolescents have demonstrated prevailing misconceptions about the ways in which HIV infection can spread. The surveys also suggest that many sexually active adolescents may neglect protecting themselves in spite of adequate knowledge.[41] Thus, there is an urgent need for intervention at a young age with accurate and comprehensible information and appropriate counseling.

HIV were to occur. How fast this increase occurs will depend on factors such as widespread use of AZT or other antivirals that slow progression of the disease and may prolong survival.[43] Moreover, improvements in therapy that prolong the survival of AIDS patients would increase the prevalence of AIDS in the population.

Future projections of the AIDS epidemic in the original epicenters vary by region. In San Francisco, where the epidemic has affected primarily homosexual White men and there is evidence of reductions in high-risk behaviors, the rate of new AIDS cases occurring per year is expected to peak by the mid-1990s and slowly decline thereafter.[44] In the Northeast, notably New York and New Jersey, where the epidemic has become primarily a disease of injection drug users and their sexual partners and offspring, the infection is spreading more rapidly, although the incidence of new infections in the general population is quite low even there.

PUBLIC HEALTH IMPLICATIONS

Modes of Transmission

In order to transmit the infection, HIV has to get from an infected individual into the bloodstream of an uninfected individual. This is known to occur in three ways: through sexual activity (where semen or vaginal fluids are passed from one individual to another), perinatally from an infected mother to her newborn and through direct transfer of infected blood. No new modes of transmission have emerged in nine years of careful epidemiologic study. The efficiency of transmission via each of these routes appears to be variable and may depend on a number of cofactors. HIV can be transmitted either as cell-free virus or in HIV-infected cells; the minimum amount of virus or number of infected cells required for transmission is unknown.[45]

SEXUAL TRANSMISSION

Epidemiologic studies of homosexual men have shown that their highest risk of acquiring HIV infection is through receptive anal intercourse, with an infected person inserting his penis into the anus of an uninfected partner.[46] The risk of transmission through insertive anal intercourse (when an uninfected person inserts his penis into the anus of an infected partner) appears to be lower, but has not been well documented. A number of sexual practices have been identified that can cause or enhance damage or weakening of the rectal mucosa and thereby facilitate transmission of HIV during anal intercourse.[47]

Normal mucosa (the membranes lining body openings such as the vagina and mouth) appears to provide an effective barrier against HIV, so that the efficiency of HIV transmission by sexual intercourse is considerably lower than for other sexually transmitted diseases such as gonorrhea, syphilis or hepatitis.[48] The size of the viral dose necessary to transmit the infection is not known, and there is little information on the factors that might modify transmissibility of the virus or a person's susceptibility to becoming infected.[49] There is speculation that infectivity may be higher during the acute syndrome in the first few weeks of infection, and there is evidence to suggest that infectivity is higher in the final stages of HIV disease[50] and in the presence of damaged skin or mucosal membranes that provide a portal of entry for the virus.[51]

There is ample epidemiologic evidence of HIV transmission through vaginal intercourse. In the United States, the infectivity of vaginal intercourse is low, so that the likelihood of acquiring HIV from an infected person through a single act of unprotected (i.e., no condom) vaginal intercourse is very low, on the order of 1 in 500.[52] This risk is estimated by studying discordant couples (one partner infected) and determining the proportion of uninfected partners who seroconvert over time. Male-to-female infectivity is probably greater than female-to-male. Some studies in the United States have found a surprisingly low cumulative likelihood of a woman becoming infected after hundreds of episodes of unprotected vaginal intercourse with an infected partner.[53] Caution must be exercised in interpreting this finding, as infection rates have differed among groups studied,[54] and the risk of becoming infected may vary among individuals.[55]

The risk of acquiring HIV infection through vaginal intercourse has been estimated according to the partner's risk group and is reported in Table 5.[56] If the partner is not in a high-risk group, the risk per sexual encounter is extremely low, even if no condom is used (1

Table 5. RISK OF HIV* INFECTION FOR HETEROSEXUAL INTERCOURSE *in the United States*

Risk Category of Partner	Assumptions			Estimated Risk of Infection	
	Prevalence of HIV Infection	Infectivity†	Condom/ Spermicide Failure Rate	1 Sexual Encounter‡	500 Sexual Encounters§
HIV serostatus unknown					
Not in any high-risk group					
Using condoms	0.0001	0.002	0.1	1 in 50,000,000	1 in 110,000
Not using condoms	0.0001	0.002	...	1 in 5,000,000	1 in 16,000
High-risk groups¶				1 in 100,000	1 in 210
Using condoms	0.05 to 0.5	0.002	0.1	to 1 in 10,000	to 1 in 21
Not using condoms	0.05 to 0.5	0.002	...	1 in 10,000 to 1 in 1,000	1 in 32 to 1 in 3
HIV seronegative					
No history of high-risk behavior#				1 in 5,000,000,000	1 in 11,000,000
Using condoms	0.000001	0.002	0.1	1 in	1 in
Not using condoms	0.000001	0.002	...	500,000,000	1,600,000
Continuing high risk behavior#					
Using condoms	0.01	0.002	0.1	1 in 500,000	1 in 1,100
Not using condoms	0.01	0.002	...	1 in 50,000	1 in 160
HIV seropositive					
Using condoms	1.0	0.002	0.1	1 in 5,000	1 in 11
Not using condoms	1.0	0.002	...	1 in 500	2 in 3

* HIV indicates human immunodeficiency virus.

†The value 0.002 represents an upper limit on the probability that an infected male will transmit HIV to an uninfected female during one episode of penile-vaginal intercourse with ejaculation. Female-to-male infectivity may be lower, and infectivity for anal intercourse or intercourse when genital ulcers are present may be higher. The value is a group mean and may vary among individuals.

‡The risk of infection for one encounter is the product of the values in columns 3 through 4 of the Table ("Assumptions").

§The risk of infection for 500 encounters is column 2 x [1 - (1 - column 3 x column 4)^{500}].

¶High-risk groups with prevalences of HIV infection at the higher end of the range given include homosexual or bisexual men and intravenous drug users from major metropolitan areas, and hemophiliacs. Groups with prevalences at the lower end of the range include homosexual or bisexual men and intravenous drug users from other parts of the country, female prostitutes, heterosexuals from countries where heterosexual spread of HIV is common (including Haiti and central Africa) and recipients of multiple blood transfusions between 1983 and 1985 from areas with a high prevalence of HIV infection.

#High-risk behavior consists of sexual intercourse or needle sharing with a member of one of the high-risk groups.

Reprinted with permission from *JAMA* Vol. 259 No. 16 (April 22/29, 1988): 2428-32. Copyright 1988 American Medical Association.

in 5 million). However, if the partner is in a high-risk group, the risk of becoming infected increases substantially, by about four orders of magnitude, while using a condom can reduce this risk by only one order of magnitude. Thus, one's risk of acquiring HIV infection through sexual intercourse depends most of all on the likelihood that one's partner is infected, and secondarily on condom use.[57]

The presence of HIV-infected cells in genital fluids may play a major role in the sexual transmission of the infection.[58] Transmission of HIV infection by artificial insemination with sperm from an infected donor has been reported.[59] Studies in Africa, where heterosexual intercourse is the major route of HIV spread, have shown that genital ulcers favor transmission, as does lack of circumcision in the male.[60] HIV has been isolated from secretions caused by tissue inflammation surrounding genital ulcers of infected persons.[61] The presence of inflammatory cells in genital ulcerations provides both a source of HIV and a site for viral entry.[62] Genital lesions may contribute to the high rate of HIV seropositivity observed in patients attending sexually transmitted disease clinics in the United States (5 percent in one recent study).[63]

A few instances of HIV transmission by oro-genital contact have been reported,[64] but whether infection can occur by this route remains controversial. The risk associated with this activity appears to be low.

BLOOD-BORNE TRANSMISSION

Transfusion of a single unit of blood from an infected donor carries a high likelihood of transmitting the infection, on the order of 80 to 90 percent.[65] However, mandatory serotesting of donors instituted in 1985, combined with rejection of potential donors who acknowledge having any risk factors, has made the risk of acquiring HIV infection via transfusion very low. The odds of acquiring HIV infection from a single unit of transfused blood have recently been estimated to be 1 in 153,000 (ranging from 1 in 88,000 to 1 in 300,000).[66] Most of this risk derives from blood donors who do not acknowledge having risk factors and who have not yet seroconverted because their infection is recent.[67]

In a recent report of blood donors in Washington, D.C., tested between July 1985 and December 1988,[68] the frequency of positive Western blot results fell from 0.14 to 0.04 percent over the 42-month study period, probably due to prior risk factor screening. Of the confirmed HIV-positive donors enrolled in the study, all were subsequently found to have identifiable risk factors. But 26 percent did not believe themselves to be at risk because they had recently changed their behavior, and another 26 percent presented for donating in order to obtain an HIV test. Another 15 percent had felt pressured into donating by family or friends and yielded to this pressure because they wanted to keep their risk factor confidential.

Patients with hemophilia or other coagulation disorders require repeated injections with coagulation factor concentrates made from pooled blood of thousands of donors. This intensity of exposure implied a high risk of infection prior to the institution of heat treatment of the concentrates in 1985; the risk of infection has substantially decreased since then.[69] Follow-up studies of patients with hemophilia have documented which decontamination methods of factor concentrates are the most effective, so that the risk of HIV infection can be expected to decrease even further.[70]

Virus may be transmitted by needle sharing among injection drug users. In drug use, blood is drawn into the syringe prior to injection to assure that the needle is in a vein, and sufficient blood often remains in the syringe to infect subsequent users.[71] HIV infection in injection drug users provides the principal mode of transmission of HIV to the heterosexual adult population and to infants through perinatal infection.[72] Inadequately sterilized parenteral material used for medical procedures or in ritual scarification (e.g., tattooing) may also transmit the infection.

Accidental inoculation of infected blood in health-care workers by needle stick or via abraded skin appears to carry a relatively small risk of infection, about 0.5 percent per exposure.[73] Although this risk is small, it represents a serious occupational hazard that can be reduced, but not completely eliminated, by taking universal precautions and treating the body fluids of every patient as potentially infected.

PERINATAL TRANSMISSION

Perinatal transmission of HIV from an infected mother to her infant has been well documented and accounts for over 80 percent of pediatric AIDS cases in the United States. HIV may be transmitted to the fetus both early and late during pregnancy,[74] and there is evidence that transmission may occur by direct infection of placental tissues.[75] Infection could also occur during the birthing process, but this does not appear to be a common path; Cesarean section has not been shown to be protective.[76] Breast milk has transmitted HIV infection in several well-documented cases of women who became infected via post-partum blood transfusions, and virus has been isolated from breast milk in both free and cellular form.[77] The efficiency of HIV transmission via breast milk is probably low and may be facilitated by breaks in the infant's mucosa, but little information is currently available.

Infants of infected mothers have maternal antibodies in their bloodstream that persist for many months after birth, but only about one-third of these infants are infected.[78] Thus, diagnosis of HIV infection in infants younger than 15 months of age cannot rely on serotesting, but must be made on a clinical basis or by using a research laboratory to detect viral components in the infants' blood. Little is known about risk factors that may enhance the rate of perinatal transmission or about interventions to prevent transmission of the infection to the infant.

HOW HIV IS NOT TRANSMITTED

There is strong epidemiologic evidence that HIV infection does not occur through intact skin; the virus can only pass through breaks in the skin or by needle puncture. HIV is not transmitted by touching, hugging, handshaking, sharing eating utensils, sneezing or sharing close living quarters.[79] Numerous studies in the United States and elsewhere have examined the risk of HIV infection in hundreds of close household contacts of both infected adults and children over many years, and no instances of HIV transmission were found.[80] Exposures included sharing of items used in personal grooming, even toothbrushes in some instances, and yet no HIV infection was found in the household contacts, except in sex partners and infants born to infected mothers.

Exchange of saliva has not been documented to transmit the infection. In the absence of blood, HIV is present in saliva in minute quantities only.[81] Close follow-up of health-care workers bitten by AIDS patients and of children bitten by HIV-infected children shows no evidence of seroconversion.[82] Thus, if close household contact does not transmit the infection, it is even less likely that HIV can be acquired by routine contact with infected persons in schools or at the work place.

HIV is not transmitted by insect bites. There is no biologic evidence supporting the hypothesis of insects as vectors of HIV transmission.[83] Moreover, the epidemiologic pattern of HIV disease is incompatible with transmission by insects: Most infected persons are 20-49 years of age; there is no reason for biting insects to display such age selectivity.

While the modes of transmission are now well understood, much work remains to be done to explain the variability in the efficiency of transmission observed in each of these modes. However, given the modes of transmission, it is clear that the propagation of the HIV epidemic depends on individual behaviors, and that further spread can be halted by changes in individual behavior and community norms.

Preventing HIV Infection

Epidemiologic evidence has identified the behavior-related modes of HIV transmission, so that risk groups can be defined on the basis of activities that put their members at risk of transmitting or acquiring the infection (Table 2). The next step, designing programs for preventing the spread of HIV, has two important aspects. First, there are policies that must be implemented, such as protecting the blood supply from contamination. But most of the preventive efforts must be focused on modifying the behaviors that carry risk of acquiring HIV infection. Approaches need to be developed for disseminating accurate, up-to-date information to help people recognize what constitutes a risk factor and to help them minimize their risk by changing their own behaviors.

Table 6 summarizes recommendations for preventing the spread of HIV infection by reducing risk factors in five settings: sexual activity, injection drug use, pregnancy and birth, medical use of blood products, and health-care practice. Risk may also vary with geographic location, such as longterm residence after 1975 in communities or countries with high HIV prevalence, for example in countries of the African malaria belt. Persons who have doubts about their own risk or that of a past or present sexual partner may wish to discuss their situation with their health-care provider; they can also seek anonymous or confidential HIV-antibody testing to clarify their HIV status. The following sections will discuss prevention in detail.

PREVENTING SEXUAL TRANSMISSION

As discussed in the previous section, the highest risk of sexual transmission is associated with anal intercourse, while vaginal intercourse carries a lower risk. The risk associated with either activity is higher for the receptive partner and is enhanced by the presence of genital lesions, by an advanced stage of disease progression and probably also by lack of circumcision. While some persons may remain uninfected in spite of a large number of unprotected sexual contacts, others may become infected after one single encounter; why such differences exist is not known. The risk of becoming infected is reduced by using latex condoms (not those made of animal tissue). Oil-based lubricants should be avoided in conjunction with condoms because they damage latex; instead, water-based gels should be used for lubrication. Although it is possible that the risk is further reduced if condoms are used in association with nonoxynol-9, a spermicidal cream that has been shown to kill HIV in the laboratory, there is no direct evidence concerning its effectiveness in real life, and the cream may cause mucosal irritation if used frequently. Condom use offers about 90 percent protection,[84] because of problems with condom breakage or user error.

The risk of acquiring HIV through sexual relations depends on the probability that the partner is infected and on the precautions taken during sexual activity.[85] For individuals who are not members of a high-risk group, carefully choosing a partner at low risk of carrying HIV is the most important preventive measure. This measure involves taking the time and effort to get to know a prospective partner

---

Table 6. PREVENTING HIV INFECTION

---

1. To prevent the sexual spread of HIV

    a. Encourage individuals to evaluate their own risk status and that of their sexual partner(s). (See text for specifics.)

    b. For individuals who have one or more of the risk factors cited in the text and are unsure of their risk status, recommend voluntary anonymous or confidential HIV-antibody testing with follow-up counseling at least six months after the occurrence of the last risk.

    c. For individuals who are HIV positive or continuing to engage in risk behaviors:
       (i) Recommend avoiding anal and vaginal sexual intercourse (safest) or
       (ii) using condoms when they do have intercourse.

    d. For individuals who are HIV negative and do not engage in any risk behaviors:
       (i) Recommend discussing HIV risk reduction with any sexual partner.
       (ii) If the partner is HIV positive or of unknown serostatus, recommend:
          • avoiding anal and vaginal sexual intercourse (safest) or
          • using condoms when they do have intercourse.

2. To prevent HIV spread by injection drug use

    a. Advise against injection drug use and recommend participation in injection drug treatment programs, if feasible.

    b. For those who continue to inject drugs, recommend:
       (i) that they not share needles or other injection equipment, and
       (ii) that they use bleach to sterilize all injection equipment.

3. To prevent perinatal spread of HIV

    a. For women who are pregnant or contemplating pregnancy and are unsure of their HIV status, recommend voluntary anonymous or confidential HIV-antibody testing with follow-up counseling. If positive, obtain counseling concerning:
       (i) deferral of pregnancy;
       (ii) termination of a current pregnancy;
       (iii) planning for mother's and infant's care, if pregnancy is continued.

    b. Advise HIV-positive mothers not to breast feed their infants. (See text.)

4. To prevent HIV spread by medical use of blood products
Dissuade high-risk persons from donating blood, screen donated blood for HIV antibodies, sterilize clotting factors and avoid unnecessary transfusions.

5. To prevent HIV infection of health-care providers
Train health-care personnel and equip facilities to promote universal precautions, i.e., to handle the body fluids of every patient as if that individual were infected with HIV.

---

well. Whenever there is doubt, the safest option is to defer sexual intercourse until the partner's risk status has been clarified and a blood test for HIV antibodies has been obtained. If intercourse is not deferred, using barrier methods of protection, such as condoms, will greatly reduce but not eliminate risk of infection.[86]

Unprotected sexual intercourse is safe in a mutually monogamous relationship between known uninfected partners or partners of long duration (at least ten years). It is also safe in a mutually monogamous relationship of shorter duration if both partners either have no history of risk behaviors or if the risk behavior was remote and a recent blood test reveals no HIV antibodies. Having sex with a partner who does not belong to a high-risk group and has had only a few long-term relationships in the past ten years carries little risk of HIV infection, about 1 in 5 million per sexual encounter, even if no condoms are used.[87] Over several years this risk would accumulate to about 1 in 16,000 (Table 5). Although this risk is still small, a long-term relationship warrants frank discussions about risk reduction measures and options for anonymous or confidential serotesting. Individuals who have doubt about their own HIV status should have access to anonymous or confidential serotesting and consider either abstaining from sex or using condoms in the meantime.

Condom use is essential in sexual intercourse with a high-risk partner. Searching for a partner who is likely to be uninfected within a risk group may not be practicable, particularly if seroprevalence is high. However, if the sexual partner in a potential long-term relationship has engaged in high-risk behaviors for HIV infection or has a history of having a sexually transmitted disease or of having many sexual partners, frank discussions concerning risk reduction practices are essential, including the option of serotesting six months after stopping high-risk behaviors. Engaging in sex with an injection drug user or with an individual who practices exchanging sex for drugs or money may carry considerable risk, because the high-risk behavior is likely to be ongoing or recurrent.[88]

Persons who are infected can use latex condoms to protect their uninfected partner, but over several years of relations the risk of transmitting HIV increases to about 1 in 11, even with condoms.[89] It would be safer to practice sexual activities that avoid ejaculating into a body cavity or onto damaged skin.[90] The use of condoms may also be desirable if both partners are infected, since it is possible that reinfection hastens progression of the disease. There is no direct evidence, but it is possible that reinfection with HIV may act like any other infectious disease agent, i.e., challenge the immune system into action and thereby induce infected immune cells to multiply and produce numerous copies of HIV (see Chapter 1).

Availability of latex condoms with instructions concerning their correct application is essential in efforts to prevent the sexual spread of HIV infection. Whenever there is a possibility that a sexual partner may be infected, intercourse should not take place without a condom. Although condoms have a failure rate of about 10 percent, they reduce the risk considerably. Even incorrect application of a condom is better than no condom use at all in situations where there is doubt. Moreover, condoms offer protection against the spread of other sexually transmitted diseases.

Finally, in order to prevent the sexual spread of HIV infection, it is important to avoid abuse of substances that impair judgment, such as alcohol or cocaine or other illicit drugs, since high-risk sexual practices may be more likely under the influence of drugs

PREVENTING TRANSMISSION THROUGH INJECTION DRUG USE

Preventing the spread of HIV via injection drug use is difficult, since it is often hard to reach injection drug users and gain their compliance with prevention efforts. There are too few detoxification programs for injection drug users who want to stop using drugs, and programs designed to help injection drug users stop sharing needles and syringes have inadequate public support and funding. For those who will continue to inject drugs, prevention strategies should include regular access to sterile injection equipment, including needle exchange programs. There is need for further intervention to reduce sexual risk behavior among injection drug users. Without such programs the risk of new infection remains high in injection drug users, their sexual partners and their children.

PREVENTING TRANSMISSION THROUGH BLOOD AND BLOOD PRODUCTS

The strategy for preventing HIV transmission by transfusion of blood and blood products uses a combination of voluntary deferral of high-risk donors and mandatory HIV serotesting. Since serology can detect HIV antibodies only after they have developed, serotesting does not help screen out blood of individuals with recently acquired infection. Risk assessment and self-deferral of potential donors are therefore very important. Some individuals presenting for blood donation do not acknowledge having past risk factors, because they have recently changed their behavior and/or because they desire HIV testing.[91] There is a great need to impart a clear, unmistakable prevention message and to persuade individuals who want to know their antibody status to use the widely available and often free anonymous or confidential serotesting programs, instead of presenting for blood donor testing.

Individuals preparing for elective surgical procedures have the option of donating blood for their own use at the time of surgery (autologous transfusion). The practice of requesting blood donations from friends or acquaintances may not be in the patient's best interest. An individual may feel pressured into donating in spite of knowing of some risk factor that he or she wants to keep confidential. In an effort to counteract this pressured-donor effect, blood banks give donors several chances to label the blood confidentially and unobtrusively as ineligible for use.

PREVENTING PERINATAL TRANSMISSION

Preventing perinatal HIV transmission requires that prospective mothers present for risk assessment and counseling prior to pregnancy or during prenatal care. Those who think they might have been infected with HIV should be advised to seek voluntary (anonymous or confidential) HIV serotesting. If the HIV test is positive, they should receive counseling concerning their options, such as deferral of pregnancy, termination of a current pregnancy or planning for the future care of their infant. HIV-infected mothers should be advised not to breastfeed their infants; the only exception to this rule should be based on the inability to provide adequate alternative nutrition, as may be the case in a developing country, where malnutrition threatens the lives of all infants and would also hasten the demise of those who are HIV-infected.

PREVENTING OCCUPATIONAL TRANSMISSION

Preventing accidental infection of health care workers is an important challenge. Although less than 0.5 percent of health-care workers have been reported to seroconvert after needlestick inoculation with HIV-infected blood (compared with up to 20 percent seroconverting after needlestick exposure to hepatitis B virus), there is as yet no proven prophylaxis for HIV infection (as there is for hepatitis B); however, some health care institutions have begun experimental use of post-exposure prophylaxis with AZT.[92] Taking universal precautions as if every patient were potentially infected may reduce but cannot eliminate this occupational hazard.[93]

Social and Cultural Prevention Issues

The future of the epidemic in any community, even in low-prevalence regions, will depend to some extent on the presence of behaviorally vulnerable groups in which HIV is likely to spread rapidly once it has been introduced. It will also depend on the success of community efforts to help these groups implement effective behavioral prevention. This section focuses on psychosocial and sociocultural aspects that may impede or foster prevention efforts and underlines the importance of having group members take a lead in HIV prevention within their communities.

THE ROLE OF THE COMMUNITY

Risk behaviors at the individual level are intimately linked with social and cultural aspects of the community in which they occur. Anonymous and multiple-partner sexual behavior among gay men in the years prior to the HIV epidemic, for example, was often consistent with gay community norms and served to strengthen and enhance gay identity.[94] Similarly, ritualistic needle sharing among injection drug users in some East Coast communities has been described as a symbol of trust and a means of bonding within the subculture.[95] In these and other ways, risk behaviors practiced by individuals reflect personal, emotional, political and economic attributes of the community. Consequently, the most powerful prevention strategies are those grounded in an understanding of cultural issues within the community and those that involve the target community in changing individual behaviors and group norms.

The response of gay men in San Francisco to the HIV epidemic is a forceful demonstration of community action applied to the problem of HIV prevention. Annual HIV seroconversion rates in this community decreased from 18 percent in 1982 to 1 percent in 1987,[96] and this decrease was accompanied by large and stable changes in sexual risk behavior. Prevention efforts relied on community-based approaches and volunteer organizations to change social norms related to sexual practices, encouraging safe sex as an alternative to high-risk practices.[97] Interventions included education about risk and risk reduction, anonymous antibody testing, media saturation with HIV-related information, organized public meetings and forums and informal small groups conducted in private homes.[98] Taken together, these strategies represent a community-level intervention of massive proportions.[99] The experience of the gay community in San Francisco indicates that HIV infection is preventable, that risk-related community norms are an achievable target for change and that the community itself is a prevention weapon. This experience, however, cannot be generalized directly to injection drug-using communities or to Black and Hispanic communities affected by the epidemic.

As discussed above, seroprevalence rates in some East Coast drug–using communities exceed 50 percent.[100] In Manhattan, for example, seroprevalence among injection drug users reached nearly 60 percent in 1984, before leveling off due to risk reduction among injection drug users and HIV saturation among those at risk.[101] In San Francisco, lower seroprevalence rates of 10-15 percent[102] indicate that saturation in the injection drug-using community has not been reached. This saturation may be avoided through aggressive prevention efforts. To this end, prevention strategies using multiple points of entry into the substance-abusing community were initiated, including clinic-based small group psychoeducational programs, clinic-based outreach to injection drug users and their sexual partners, street outreach to addicts not in treatment and an unsanctioned needle exchange program.

Injection drug users responded to prevention efforts by taking steps to decrease infection risk. The use of bleach to disinfect needles increased dramatically between 1985 and 1987,[103] and needle-sharing behavior has decreased over time.[104] Preliminary serologic data suggest that annual seroconversion rates also declined, from 7 percent in 1985 to slightly over 2 percent in 1987.[105] Unlike the gay community, however, the needle-using community lacked the infrastructure, self-organization[106] and political and financial power necessary to implement multiple prevention programs. Leadership in HIV prevention came not from within the drug-using community, but from ex-addicts, addiction counselors and health care providers and public health professionals, most of whom previously served the injection drug-using community.

The HIV epidemic is also a Black and Hispanic epidemic, and there continues to be a great need for prevention programs targeting Black and Hispanic persons at risk. These communities face unique challenges in developing effective HIV prevention programs. Minority gay men, for example, may perceive their risk of infection to be lower than it is, may be isolated from prevention messages for cultural reasons and may have fewer formal gay organizations to act as conduits for behavior change information.[107] Community-based organizations in minority communities may feel overwhelmed by current service demands, may lack the resources necessary to carry out a new prevention mission and may fear the political fallout attendant to active involvement in HIV prevention.[108] Further, AIDS cannot easily rise to the top of the agenda, because many ethnic minority communities experience the epidemic in the context of multiple social problems, such as drug use, poverty, crime and inadequate health care, that result from their status as marginalized groups.[109]

MARGINALIZATION AND ITS EFFECTS

Discrimination has created subcultures that are barred from full participation in society's social, political and economic systems, thus marginalizing these subcultural groups. Since homosexuals, injection drug users and Blacks and Hispanics are among the hardest hit by HIV disease, marginalization critically affects the course of the epidemic. It delays response to the epidemic, encourages denial of it and prompts overreactions to HIV that often blame the ill and endanger public health.[110] Thus, halting the HIV epidemic depends upon the ability to understand and interrupt the effects of marginalization.

For Blacks and Hispanics, marginalization has meant depressed socioeconomic status and political disenfranchisement. Roughly one in three Blacks and Hispanics live below poverty level. Seventy-nine percent of Blacks and 58 percent of Hispanics have a high school education, and 13 percent and 10 percent hold college degrees. Blacks and Hispanics experience unemployment at nearly twice the rate of Whites, and the Black mortality rate is 1.5 times that of Whites.[111] While Blacks and Hispanics represent nearly 20 percent of the United States population, they are just 3 percent of elected officials.[112]

Society's view of marginalized groups is often clouded by prejudice. The true identities of marginalized people may be superseded by the collective image the dominant culture has created for them. Legitimate differences in language, custom and culture mingle with artificial differences to justify oppression or to simplify a confusing cultural diversity. As a result, ignorance and antipathy guide the conceptualization of AIDS as a disease of specific, undesirable groups, thus delaying recognition of the disease and obstructing the development of effective prevention efforts.[113] In addition, social prejudices have made this epidemic the most political of epidemics in recent history.[114]

Black and Hispanic communities have been slow to embrace AIDS as their issue not only because of limited resources and the cultural biases against homosexuality and illicit drug use, but also because they do not wield the political clout to protect themselves against the additional stigma that AIDS brings. In addition, they have been suspicious of intervention coming from outside their ethnic communities.

It has been said many times that HIV prevention efforts must be culturally specific to target audiences. It is equally important, however, for such programs to take into account the social history of the marginalized people they hope to serve. Distrust and ignorance exist on both sides of the barriers that hem in members of marginalized groups. When fear is introduced, as it is in the HIV epidemic, an impasse may arise that can halt efforts to mobilize against the epidemic. Fear of AIDS takes on many forms: fear of illness, powerlessness, stigma, and of death, dying, sexuality, drug use, discrimination.[115]

It is in this complex network that the spread of HIV disease must be halted. Those who are believed to be vastly different or "deviant" must be approached with respect and an eagerness to learn from them in order to understand how best to teach them. The task is one of building bridges over social barriers, because marginalization and the resulting fear and ignorance are problems of long standing with no easy solutions.

SUMMARY

Public health and medical authorities are mandated to protect the public from risk beyond individual control by assuring the safety of medical practices via strict mandatory blood and organ donor screening for HIV antibody and for risk factors. Beyond this mandate, public health decision makers have an important role as facilitators of voluntary behavior changes on an individual and group level.

Individuals who are not infected need to know how to protect themselves by avoiding behaviors associated with risk. Those who are infected need to be able to find out that they are infected, without fear of recrimination, and to change their behaviors, both to prevent transmission of their infection to others and to protect themselves against reinfection. Behavior change is the effective means of preventing further spread of HIV. It will always be a major thrust, even when effective biomedical prophylaxis or a curative treatment become available, because the use of a vaccine or a curative treatment alone cannot be expected to stop a behaviorally mediated epidemic. The evidence for this is the persistence of hepatitis B, despite the availability of a safe and effective vaccine, and the resurgence of syphilis, despite effective antibiotics.

Community leaders and their agencies must take stock of their constituencies. The behavioral prevention message must be cast in an explicit language that is adapted to each particular culture and delivered by persons that the group will accept. Voluntary behavior change must be facilitated by designing interventions that take into account the particular needs of each group in a nonjudgmental manner. Safeguards are necessary to block prejudice from interfering with effective preventive measures. An enlightened community will enlist the support of those who are infected by creating accessible and safe services for voluntary anonymous or confidential testing, by preventing discrimination and by providing appropriate counseling while providing medical care.

Thus, the role of public health leaders includes the provision of accurate information about the disease and how it spreads, the prevention of discrimination and other prejudicial measures and the provision of resources and tools needed to bring about behavior change.

AIDS:
Putting the Models to the Test

Margaret A. Chesney
and Thomas J. Coates

INTRODUCTION

Over the course of this century, life expectancy in the United States has increased by 50 percent.[1] In 1900 males had an expected life of 48.2 years at birth, while females were expected to live 51.1 years.[2] By contrast, in the 1980s, males are expected to live 70.8 years, while females can be expected to live 78.2 years.[3] In this chapter, the reasons for this remarkable increase in longevity will be examined. The evolutionary changes in health promotion and illness prevention will also be discussed, placing programs directed toward HIV risk reduction in an historical and theoretical context. The objective of this chapter is to increase awareness of the history of health promotion, so HIV prevention efforts can benefit from previous lessons learned.

Health promotion and disease prevention, as they are known today, were not the driving forces behind the nation's improving health during most of this century. Since the 1970s, however, health promotion efforts, buttressed by the new field of behavioral medicine, have demonstrated significant health benefits. Perhaps the most impressive of these benefits has been the reduction in cardiovascular risk, which has been reflected in a notable decline in coronary heart disease.[4] Led by the National High Blood Pressure Education Program, the federal government launched blood pressure screening campaigns that identified hypertensive individuals, referred them for care and taught them the importance of adhering to treatment. These efforts have been credited with a marked improvement in detection, treatment and control of hypertension across the country. Specifically, in the 1970s, approximately 50 percent of those with elevated blood pressure were unaware of their condition. By 1980 this number had dropped to 27 percent.[5] Over the decade 1970 to 1980, the proportion of people with hypertension who had controlled their blood pressure more than doubled to 34 percent from 16 percent, and reports from surveys conducted between 1982 and 1984 put this figure at 57 percent.[6]

During the last two decades, Americans also made major changes in their diets,[7] which corresponded with significant decreases in the nation's cholesterol levels.[8] The benefits of these and other changes in cardiovascular risk factors, including sharp reductions in the percentage of Americans who smoke cigarettes, have been demonstrated in randomized clinical trials, epidemiological studies and clinical observations.[9]

With these successes as well as some failures in mind, researchers in behavioral medicine and health promotion also began discovering—and attempting to address—weaknesses in their approaches when the HIV epidemic began in the early 1980s. Thus, the recent history of health promotion and illness prevention not only provides models for programs directed at HIV risk reduction but also foretells certain arenas where HIV risk reduction may stumble or fall. Innovative concepts such as "self-efficacy," a concept that recognizes the importance of people's beliefs about their ability to successfully carry out health recommendations, extend earlier health promotion and illness prevention models and hold promise for addressing the challenge that AIDS presents to the public health of our nation and its communities.

THE GERM THEORY AND MODERN MEDICINE

The health revolution of this past century can be largely attributed to two advances. The first of these advances was the germ theory, a revolutionary concept in modern medicine that came to the fore in the late nineteenth century, focusing the health establishment's attention on the elimination of microbiological, chemical and physical causes of disease and disability from the environment.

The second advance consisted of the conceptual and technical achievements of medicine in the second half of the twentieth century. For instance, modern biochemistry has developed remarkably, increasing our understanding of the biochemical workings of the body and the pathogens that invade it. In addition, the development of vaccines and antibiotics gave medicine effective weapons against infectious diseases that formerly killed millions. The great influenza epidemic of 1918-19, for example, caused many deaths because of bacterial pneumonias. These pneumonias can now be successfully treated. Smallpox has been eliminated worldwide, and poliomyelitis, rubella and whooping cough have been virtually eliminated from the United States as a result of advances in immunology and the development of immunization science and technology.

At the same time, diagnostic procedures have improved our ability to identify a variety of diseases at earlier stages, and improvements in surgery, radiology and drug therapy have provided effective treatments for conditions that were once considered fatal and untreatable. Thus, the past century has seen a health revolution in which the major causes of death and disability in the United States shifted from infectious diseases to chronic diseases. Research on chronic diseases has revealed that each could be related, at least in part, to individual lifestyles and specific health behaviors, such as consumption of diets high in fat, physical inactivity and cigarette smoking. This realization led to a shift in public health efforts from the environment and the agent to the host—or to individual behavior.

BEHAVIOR REPLACES THE GERM AS TARGET

Since the 1960s, public health attention has turned increasingly toward designing health promotion and illness prevention programs intended to eliminate unhealthy behaviors and to prevent such diseases as coronary heart disease, cancer and stroke, our first-, second- and third-ranked killers. In 1978 then-United States Secretary of Health, Education and Welfare, Joseph Califano, called upon Americans to affirm these new challenges to the public health and to seek to ameliorate them. In a report to President Jimmy Carter, Califano wrote to each American:

> ...You, the individual, can do more for your own health and well-being than any doctor, any hospital, any exotic medical device. Indeed, a wealth of scientific research reveals that the key to whether a person will be healthy or sick, live a long life or die prematurely, can be found in several simple personal habits: One's habits with regard to smoking and drinking; one's habits of diet, sleep and exercise; whether one obeys the speed laws and wears seat belts, and a few other simple measures.[10]

Unhealthy behaviors had become the "germs" of the latter part of the twentieth century. Germ theory was joined by behavioral theories to provide the conceptual foundation for public health.

One of the first health promotion campaigns that attempted to change behavior in the United States was initiated in 1964 by the Office of the Surgeon General, which warned of the health risks associated with cigarette smoking. The Surgeon General's landmark document was the first widely publicized report linking cigarette smoking with disease.[11] Still, the warning came too late for many. For example, it was the increase in cigarette smoking among women that accounted for lung cancer taking over the lead from breast cancer as the most common cancer among women by 1986.[12] Efforts to discourage smoking have intensified since the 1964 report from general health education to direct public policy interventions, such as tobacco and alcohol tax increases, advertising bans and the restriction on or prohibition of smoking in public places.

Parallels to the earlier medical advances over infectious disease abound in the health promotion campaign against smoking. Some programs have targeted young people and even speak of "immunizing" them against initiation of smoking.[13] These programs focus on developing antismoking attitudes among children before they consider smoking. Strategies have included peer-led educational programs about health risks of smoking and structured roleplaying to teach youths to resist peer pressure for smoking. Also, paralleling the medical advances that involved eliminating pathogens from the environment came the focus on restricting cigarette smoking in public settings, which reduces the risks to nonsmokers of secondhand smoke.

CHANGING BEHAVIOR: THE FIVE STAGES

Health promotion, disease prevention and effective use of alternative methods for treating disease require that individuals change their unhealthy behaviors and that organizations be restructured to promote these efforts. Behavioral medicine emerged in the latter part of the 1970s as the field concerned with providing a scientific basis and theoretical foundation for understanding what motivates the persistence of unhealthy habits and what approaches are effective in establishing new, healthier alternatives. The push to introduce health promotion programs to address known risk factors often preceded careful testing. Thus, what happened during the 1980s in health promotion was evolution by trial and error. The scientific work of behavioral medicine often occurred independently or only as an adjunct to health promotion programs. As a result, programs did not fully benefit from scientific research, and the research findings did not readily generalize to the public health arena.

By the mid-1980s, much had been learned, and successes and failures had been documented. Most noteworthy, there was a relative lack of success in health promotion among ethnic populations, in maintenance of behavior change and in preventing the acquisition of unhealthy behaviors among youth. These problems were seen most clearly in the continued prevalence of smoking among many groups.

Specifically, the last decade shows an evolution of health promotion efforts—by trial and error—through a series of stages. Critical accounts by such leaders in the field as Lawrence Green,[14] Marshall Becker[15] and John Kirscht[16] have been integrated into what has been characterized as a series of stages. This staging also has benefited the fields of health education, health promotion, illness prevention and behavioral medicine.[17]

The *first stage* emphasizes information transfer. The provision of information often constitutes the entire health promotion effort, until it is realized that information alone is not sufficient to foster and maintain health behavior changes. The *second stage* consists of specific efforts to motivate behavior change and examines the role played by individual attitudes and beliefs about health and illness in determining whether health information will lead to new behaviors. The *third stage* introduces the importance of training, when it becomes apparent that "good" intentions do not always translate into specific plans of action; this stage promotes practical training in the skills necessary to implement intentions for a healthier lifestyle. At the *fourth stage*, it is recognized that skills must be reinforced by efforts to convey the notion that change is possible in the face of sizable difficulties and obstacles. Still, despite each of these stages and approaches, health promotion campaigns often fell short, and health behavior changes were not adopted or sustained. This has brought health promotion to the present *fifth stage*, which takes into account how environmental factors alternatively serve as barriers to, or motivators for, the introduction and maintenance of health behavior changes.

Repeating this evolutionary health promotion cycle for each illness costs valuable time. In the case of HIV disease, lost time translates into lost lives. This loss of lives is why it is important to understand what health promotion and disease prevention efforts can and cannot accomplish.

Stage 1: Providing Information
Once medicine or science identifies a behavior as a risk factor for a disease, many health professionals assume that informing the public of the risk will be sufficient to promote behavior change. The health promotion field is filled with programs that focus entirely on

giving the public factual information about risk, illness and the importance of health-enhancing behaviors. In the treatment of hypertension, for example, it has long been assumed that giving patients information about the risk of high blood pressure would increase adherence to medication schedules and other anti-hypertensive regimens. Based on this premise, blood pressure screening and education programs were implemented. These provide striking examples of the limitations of information alone in changing behavior. While the programs were effective in educating those with hypertension about their condition, the increased knowledge did not result in increased adherence to treatment or blood pressure control.[18]

Health promotion programs, often beginning with an exclusive focus on information transfer, have been expanded or redesigned time after time as it has become clear that these programs were insufficient to promote behavior changes in most individuals.

Not surprisingly, the health promotion and behavioral medicine literature would predict that information alone will be ineffective in promoting behaviors that reduce the risk of HIV transmission. As will be discussed later in this book, early research in San Francisco confirmed this prediction. As part of the AIDS Behavioral Research Project (a project of the University of California, San Francisco), a questionnaire was sent to 1,550 gay males in the San Francisco Bay Area.[19] This questionnaire asked the men for factual information about AIDS and HIV risk reduction as well as about their personal sexual practices. The study concluded that while the men were uniformly well-informed about AIDS and HIV risk-reducing practices, the information was not sufficient to foster change in their high-risk behavior. The authors wrote, "Sexual behavior may be comparable to other high-risk behaviors such as tobacco smoking, obesity, nonseat belt use and alcohol consumption, where knowledge alone is not sufficient to change behavior."[20]

AIDS education programs that rely only on providing information through posters, pamphlets or public service announcements are not likely to achieve changes in HIV risk behaviors without adding elements from the other stages of health promotion.

Stage 2: Motivation and Persuasion

The second stage in the evolution of health promotion consists of specific efforts to motivate recipients to change behavior. The most common strategy first employed to influence behavior change is fear arousal, which emphasizes the adverse consequences of failing to adopt health behaviors. A controversy over the impact of fear arousal emerged in behavioral medicine research and remains unresolved. Some argue that fear arousal increases motivation, while others contend that it leads to denial and undermines motivation to change health behavior.[21] In any case, for the evolution of health promotion, the introduction of fear arousal signaled the recognition that individual factors could influence people's responses to health information.[22] Moreover, behavioral medicine research on fear arousal demonstrated that individual factors, such as attitudes about health and beliefs about personal susceptibility to disease, can be manipulated. This knowledge led to more sophisticated models of motivation and persuasion.

Responding to this new knowledge, the Health Belief Model was proposed by researchers to integrate individual factors into a theoretical framework for health promotion. Developed by the United States Public Health Service to explain why some individuals seek preventive health services while others do not, the model was subsequently extended to a wide range of health promotion efforts.[23] In its most recent form, the general model argues that the likelihood that an individual will engage in a specific health behavior is related to beliefs about: (1) personal vulnerability to illness; (2) perceived seriousness of illness, if not prevented; (3) perceived efficacy of the recommended behaviors in reducing vulnerability; and (4) perceived costs or barriers associated with behavior change.

Among the beliefs incorporated in the Health Belief Model, two, perceived vulnerability and barriers and costs, have taken on major significance. Considerable behavioral medicine research supports their importance in determining the success of health promotion programs.[24]

PERCEIVED VULNERABILITY

Individuals' beliefs about their vulnerability or susceptibility to disease can determine whether health information is acted upon. Thus, a challenge for health promotion is personalizing health risk by conveying vulnerability. The relevance of perceived vulnerability in AIDS education has been noted by J. Weber, Thomas J. Coates and Leon McKusick,[25] who found that denial of personal risk for HIV infection was associated with high-risk sexual behavior among gay men living in San Francisco. Research with adolescents[26] has also demonstrated the pivotal importance of this belief and underscores the challenge for health promotion among young people. Specifically, research[27] has shown that adolescents often initiate and continue to engage in a high-risk or unhealthy behavior, at least in part due to their belief that any adverse impact on their actual health would occur in the distant future.

Health promotion programs and behavioral medicine research have not found an effective way to communicate personal relevance and perceived vulnerability to health risks of such addictive behaviors as smoking and drug abuse among adolescents. Thus, the health promotion literature would predict that HIV risk reduction among adolescents would also be difficult to achieve.

Costs vs. Benefits

Practitioners in the field of health promotion, health education and behavioral medicine naturally assume that individuals make decisions about performance of risky or healthy behaviors. This decision-making process has been outlined by the theoretical model of I. Ajzen and Martin Fishbein and is described as "reasoned action."[28] Specifically, this model argues that individuals make choices about new behaviors by weighing their benefits and costs. While those in health promotion often emphasize the benefits of healthy behaviors, there are also barriers and costs involved in initiating and maintaining new behaviors.

Adolescents, for example, may have the information necessary to engage in low-risk sexual behaviors to avoid contracting HIV. They may believe themselves to be vulnerable to infection if they fail to practice low-risk behaviors, and conversely, safer if they limit themselves to low-risk practices. However, they might still choose to practice high-risk behaviors because they view the potential costs of engaging in low-risk behavior, such as potential rejection from peers and sexual partners, to outweigh the possible benefits accrued in terms of reduced risk.

Health promotion research models would predict that, in order to be effective, HIV prevention program designers must recognize and address the factors that play a role in health behavior decision making, including potential psychosocial costs. According to M. Z. Solomon and W. DeJong,[29] "Unrealistic messages will lose their credibility among individuals who know firsthand the very real costs associated with changing important aspects of their lives." That such costs exist in association with behavioral risk reduction in gay men has recently been documented in the Multicenter AIDS Cohort Study.[30] These costs have included increases in psychological distress as well as increases in anxiety and depression.

Stage 3: Teaching Specific Skills

In addition to providing individuals with information and convincing them of the positive cost-benefit ratio involved in taking the recommended health action, health promotion experts have learned that it is necessary to train recipients in the specific skills required to carry out that action.[31] For example, smoking prevention programs to deter the onset of cigarette smoking in adolescents evolved to include an emphasis on social skills training for young people to teach them to anticipate and override social pressures to smoke from peers, adult models and media advertisements.

Surveys indicated that young people knew the dangers of smoking and as children had sentiments against smoking. However, as the children studied "grew older, social pressures to smoke became superimposed on the fear of this behavior, and the fear and knowledge of the danger of smoking became insufficient to prevent the onset of smoking."[32]

The importance of specific skills training has been demonstrated throughout the short history of health promotion and behavioral medicine. Programs with skills components include those designed to reduce alcohol abuse among adolescents,[33] to prevent accidents and injury in children,[34] to promote weight reduction and management[35] and to promote oral health.[36]

Health promotion literature would predict that programs that rely on arousing fear of personal vulnerability and emphasizing the protective benefits of low-risk behavior will be handicapped and perhaps ineffective in preventing HIV transmission by behavior change if they do not teach specific skills required in performance of low-risk behavior. Specifically, these skills involve practicing safe sex, cleaning hypodermic needles and most importantly, communicating with others (for example, sexual partners) whose cooperation is required to carry out risk reduction.

Stage 4: Increasing Self-Efficacy

Health promotion and behavioral medicine have a checkered past in modifying health behaviors. While hundreds of thousands of Americans have changed health habits, many of those at elevated risk (e.g., those who continue cigarette smoking or remain obese despite participation in health promotion programs) have failed to apply successfully the skills taught. In recent years, the health promotion field has evolved by incorporating the conceptual model and pioneering research of Albert Bandura.[37] This research demonstrated that perceived efficacy affects every phase of health behavior change—from whether a person even considers changing health habits to the effort exerted, the amount of change desired and even the extent to which the changes are maintained.

Perceived self-efficacy is concerned with people's beliefs about their ability to carry out a chosen health behavior and how much effort they will invest in the face of difficulties or resistance. The degree of perceived self-efficacy has been shown to be an essential variable in the adoption of new behaviors as well as in the ability to sustain health efforts. For example, cigarette smokers who perceive themselves as incapable of giving up smoking do not even try, or if they do, they are often unsuccessful, quickly abandoning their efforts regardless of the extent of their knowledge and fear concerning the health hazards of smoking.[38]

Turning to AIDS, less than one-half of sexually active Stanford University students recently surveyed used safe sex methods, and most of the students reported avoiding even discussing safe sex with their partners.[39] A survey conducted as part of the San Francisco

AIDS Behavioral Cohort Study revealed that gay and bisexual men were knowledgeable about the importance of safe sex activities to prevent HIV transmission. However, those who did not believe that they could successfully implement such practices in their relationships (i.e., those with low self-efficacy) were unable to act on their knowledge.[40]

The perceived efficacy of the behaviors in actually lowering one's risk and one's self-efficacy to engage in those behaviors were more strongly related to the practice of low-risk behaviors (i.e., safe sex) than *knowledge* about low-risk behaviors, peer support and age.

To be most effective, HIV education programs will need to influence perceptions of self-efficacy ("I can do it") and response efficacy ("This behavior change will reduce my risk"). The importance of this was illustrated in a study of 814 gay and bisexual men residing in San Francisco.[41] Questionnaires were used to examine the relationship between self-efficacy and self-report of practicing behaviors that place an individual at high risk for HIV infection. Self-efficacy and a measure of response efficacy related specifically to safe sex practices were the two variables most strongly related to self-report of risk behaviors. This finding indicates that the leading determinants of low-risk behaviors were the men's belief in their ability to perform these behaviors. Conversely, factors not related to the practice of low-risk behaviors included knowledge or information about low-risk behaviors, peer support and age.

These studies focused on HIV risk behaviors. Thus, as had been shown with health behaviors, programs to reduce behaviors that place individuals at high risk for HIV infection need to go beyond conveying knowledge, skills and vulnerability to risk. They need also to enhance the program recipient's personal efficacy regarding lower-risk behaviors.

Stage 5: Maintaining Changed Behavior

Individual choices about health and efforts to change behaviors occur in a network of social influences. As Bandura wrote, "People who are fully informed on the modes of HIV transmission and effective self-protective methods acquire the virus only if they allow it to happen. They often allow it to happen because interpersonal, sociocultural, religious and economic factors operate as constraints on self-protective behaviors."[42]

Health promotion marshaled these forces to support health behavior change in large community cardiovascular disease intervention studies.[43] Social marketing principles, such as focus group testing and the findings from knowledge, attitude, behavior and belief surveys, were applied to change social norms, to support behavior change and to create a social environment conducive to health-enhancing behaviors.[44]

The history of health promotion argues for the power such norms can exert in support of health education efforts. This power is suggested by the dramatic changes in behavior that have been observed in the gay community of San Francisco in response to aggressive community organizing and mobilization that has occurred because of the HIV epidemic. However, experience in health promotion would also argue that a continued focus on specific high-risk groups, such as gay men or injection drug users, will limit the extent to which other groups or communities will work to establish norms for low-risk behaviors. It will also maintain a false belief among members of these other social groups that they are not vulnerable to HIV infection.

Maintenance of behavior change was the primary challenge confronted by health promotion and behavioral medicine practitioners at the time that the HIV epidemic appeared. The literature is overflowing with research showing that the effects of illness prevention and health promotion decline with time.[45] This well-known phenomenon is convincingly portrayed in the areas of weight reduction[46] and smoking cessation.[47] For example, smoking intervention programs are often successful in promoting cessation, but as many as 50 to 75 percent of those who quit relapse within the first three months of followup.

The disappointing results of health promotion in terms of effective maintenance of changes forced behavioral medicine researchers to develop relapse prevention and maintenance as a field in its own right. For example, researchers studying recidivism in former smokers have discovered that patterns of relapse often occur in the face of life stress and negative mood states and are different for males and females. These findings have been interpreted as an indication that different programs may be needed for males and females. Although relapse from safe sex has been less prevalent among gay-identified men in San Francisco than these other examples of relapse,[48] the frequency with which it occurs is a matter of great concern and is currently the focus of new prevention efforts in San Francisco.

In HIV risk reduction, attention is focused on changing high-risk to low-risk behaviors. Little attention is given to the essential task of helping people continue to practice low-risk behaviors indefinitely. Therefore, programs specifically designed for enhancing the maintenance of low-risk behaviors must be designed, tested and implemented. The health promotion literature would predict that these programs will need to be tailored to different populations and in the case of adolescents, repeated as they age and transverse various stages of social development.

SUMMARY

This chapter has shown how health promotion efforts initiated in the 1970s have evolved from the simple information transfer to programs designed to enhance retention of information and maintenance of behavior change. Historically, as health promotion efforts focused on new health behaviors, public health has been slow to apply the lessons learned from health education in the past. The specter of the HIV epidemic demands that these lessons be conscientiously and rapidly incorporated in widespread HIV prevention campaigns.

With regard to HIV prevention, the historical evolution of health promotion would predict better success if the programs were to: (1) provide the most current information about prevention of HIV transmission; (2) communicate to various population groups their personal susceptibility to this devastating disease, point out the benefits of performing recommended behaviors and effectively address the fact that these same behaviors might involve personal costs; (3) teach the specific skills necessary to implement successfully the new behaviors that reduce risk of HIV infection; (4) enhance perceived self-efficacy in the implementation of these new behaviors despite difficulties; and (5) develop a cultural and social environment that is conducive to the initiation, establishment and maintenance of HIV-risk reducing behavior.

The HIV epidemic presents a challenge to the public health community that is greater than any in recent medical history. The lessons learned in recent decades about health promotion must be applied to modify both social norms and personal behaviors if prevention program designers are to be successful in effectively containing the HIV epidemic.

Part II

The San Francisco Response

A City Responds to Crisis: Creating New Approaches

Jeffery W. Amory

INTRODUCTION

Throughout the United States and in many other countries, San Francisco's overall response to the HIV epidemic has gained renown in the eyes of some policymakers, public health officials, health care providers, prevention program designers, and researchers. Frequently referred to as the "San Francisco model," the city's response includes innovations in health care delivery and support services as well as in prevention and risk-reduction programs. This chapter examines the prevention and risk-reduction aspects of the model developed from 1982 to 1989.

The term "model" is used here with some hesitation, because of the different expectations that the word engenders. It is a catchword, widely used to encompass San Francisco's response to the HIV epidemic and, as such, cannot be ignored. For some health educators and behavioral scientists, however, the term suggests cohesiveness in theory and rigor in application and evaluation. In fact, the San Francisco model is not and was never intended to be a model in this sense.

A model in this sense is typically a closely argued theoretical construct that results in a prescription for generating behavior change in a particular population group. While San Francisco's HIV prevention and risk reduction efforts have provided opportunities for a number of different interventions that would qualify as models of this sort, the general framework of San Francisco's overall effort itself meets few of the criteria established for such models (see discussion of theories and concepts of behavior change in Chapter 3). The overall effort has not, for example, been based upon a particular theoretical construct. On the contrary, prevention efforts have been driven largely by a great sense of urgency ("Something needs to be done and right away!"), a general conviction that there is no one "best buy" among the theoretical constructs available* and the assumption that a full range of approaches should be implemented simultaneously from a wide variety of bases. The hybrid "Morin model," discussed below, has provided a sense of theoretical cohesion to the overall prevention effort, but it has never driven all aspects of the effort in the way one might expect from a theoretical model.

San Francisco's overall prevention effort also departs from more rigorous models in not having been tested under very controlled circumstances. Researchers in San Francisco have undoubtedly collected more survey data of HIV-related knowledge, attitudes, beliefs and behaviors of people targeted by prevention programs and conducted more studies of patterns of HIV seroconversion than in any other locale in the country. However, while there is clear and extensive evidence showing that high-risk behaviors have been modified among targeted groups, with most of those changes sustained over time, there are no data that convincingly associate aggregate and

---

* This observation holds primarily for the generalists who work with the overall continuum of AIDS services in San Francisco. It goes almost without saying that the staff and advocates of a *specific* prevention component are often convinced that the theoretical construct of their particular program is indeed a best buy and crucial to changing the attitudes and behavior of the population they are working with.

long-term changes with specific approaches or combinations of approaches. In other words, evaluations have not been sufficiently controlled to establish what elements—other than "all" elements— are both necessary and sufficient to realize such changes in the community. The redundancy of approaches and overlap among audiences engaged by various program components are extensive enough, though, to make it likely that most residents of San Francisco have been exposed, in one way or another, to more than one prevention effort.

There are also some very persuasive statistics on changes in HIV seroconversion[1] and rectal gonorrhea[2] rates among homosexual men that suggest that many of the behavior changes promoted among gay men to prevent HIV transmission had been undertaken by many of them before the end of 1982 (i.e., before the prevention programs described in this book were implemented). These data have encouraged speculation that the most important contribution of these programs has been to support maintenance of change, rather than to initiate it.

THE THREE ELEMENTS: AUDIENCES, APPROACHES AND MESSAGES

There are three dimensions in the framework adopted by the AIDS Office of the San Francisco Department of Public Health (DPH) for San Francisco's overall prevention model: audiences, approaches and messages.[3] Every program component that has emerged since 1982 can be described and its place in the continuum clarified with reference to each of these three dimensions. The discussion that follows also identifies principles and policies that have shaped the overall prevention effort.

Audiences
Prevention programs in San Francisco frequently target a particular group or groups. Although these efforts are often discussed in terms that suggest that each program addresses a distinct audience, the groups are not mutually exclusive in many respects. In reality,

the success of an effort defined as targeting one particular audience complements and enhances other efforts that identify their audiences differently.

As San Francisco's overall prevention effort has grown, the assumption that "community" or "subculture" identity is the key to initiating or supporting behavior change has enjoyed increasing favor among policymakers as well as providers. Behavior change is the intended outcome of most of San Francisco's prevention efforts, and there is widespread conviction that such change must be fostered within an affected community by people recognized and respected as belonging to that community.

What follows is a description of the group and audience labels used by the Department of Public Health AIDS Office.

• *Groups defined by identity* are associated with circumstances of birth, heritage and/or upbringing. Frequently, such groups are referred to as "communities" or "subcultures," each with its own sense of bondedness, communication patterns and behavioral and cultural norms. Examples include groups defined by sexual orientation, gender, ethnicity, age group and inherited condition (e.g., hemophilia).

• *Groups defined by behavior* also often share a sense of bondedness, communication patterns and norms. The degree of bondedness is in many cases influenced by the extent to which individuals in the group share a sense of being alienated from the mainstream or dominant culture. These groups include men who have sex with other men,* substance abusers, injection drug users/needle sharers, people whose sexual behaviors are disinhibited by substance use, and workers in the sex industry. Other groups, such as heterosexuals with multiple or high-risk sexual partners, do not usually share a sense of community or common norms, but the behavior group definition has been a helpful designation for prevention program designers.

• *Groups defined by location or setting* are often targeted by health educators because they provide readily identifiable audiences. Examples of groups identified by their availability for interventions in certain settings or locations include: consumers of health care services, prison inmates, youth in school, employees of the same com-

---

* The label "men who have sex with other men" is used to include not only men identifying as gay or bisexual but those who act as such while maintaining a heterosexual self-identification.

pany, members of a church, community groups or social organizations and residents of a particular neighborhood.

• *Groups defined by other circumstances* that are unique to the modes of HIV transmission include people who might have been infected through receipt of blood transfusions or use of blood products or those occupationally at risk, such as health care workers. These are not behavior groups; nevertheless, the group association may put group members' partners at risk through sexual behavior.

• *People who are already infected by HIV* and whose prevention agenda includes limiting the progress to clinical disease (i.e., secondary prevention) are an emerging audience for early intervention programs.

The "general public" is a term that has been used with different meanings in conjunction with HIV prevention. The term is sometimes used to mean "everyone." Other times, it means "everyone not at high risk." At still other times, it means "only those not in a classically defined 'high-risk group'" (i.e., someone other than men who have sex with men and injection drug users), but individuals whose behavior may still put them at risk. It is important to prevention efforts that the general public, even those at low risk, understand the general dimensions of the epidemic and the complexity and potential costs of prevention programs (in terms of lives and dollars), so that support for constructive and cost-effective interventions will be forthcoming.

Approaches

The following list of approaches was initially drafted by the San Francisco Department of Public Health AIDS Office in 1984 to encompass the sum of prevention efforts in the city. The approaches are listed in an order that reflects increasing individual involvement and confrontation. Each program in the prevention/risk-reduction continuum utilizes one or more of the following general approaches to promote awareness and/or support behavior change:

• media advertising
• news and feature coverage in print and electronic media
• materials development/product distribution
• telephone information and referral

• forums, workshops, classes and other one-time small group encounters
  • individual health education and counseling
  • interactive peer groups

No one approach is considered to be sufficient or fully independent of any other approach, and no one provider is expected to use all approaches. Within a community, however, all approaches are expected to be in play at the same time.

In San Francisco, different providers have taken responsibility for approaching particular audiences. The design of each program component may vary dramatically from one provider to another and also may vary among audiences targeted. Campaigns using a variety of approaches have been undertaken to target a specific population group with a loosely or tightly coordinated effort. For example, "Black people get AIDS, too!" became the theme of a campaign that included media advertising, pamphlets and videos from one provider; news and feature stories, street outreach and workshops, and individual health education and counseling were organized by another provider.

Messages

General concepts regarding what prompts and enables people to change their behavior and to maintain the changes were developed by an ad hoc community task force convened in early 1984. This effort became the first step in developing a long-range HIV prevention plan in the city. Since then, these concepts have been informally referred to as the "Morin model," named after San Francisco psychologist Steve Morin, who reviewed the literature on behavior change and synthesized important theoretical concepts for the task force. In brief, Morin's review identified five generic beliefs that are typically engaged when behavior change is successfully undertaken by an individual. These beliefs have a generic expression and an AIDS-specific expression. These expressions are often referred to as the underlying messages of campaigns or activities.

  • *Perceived risk*: "AIDS is a threat to me."
  • *Response efficacy*: "AIDS can be avoided."
  • *Personal or self-efficacy*: "I am capable of making the changes

necessary to avoid AIDS."
  • *Social skills*: "I am capable of communicating limits to others."
  • *Peer support*: "The norms of my community (the community group I identify with most closely) support these new behaviors."

When the *overall prevention effort* was first described in terms consistent with the Morin model, a few health educators who had developed *specific components* based on other academic models expressed discomfort with his description. It eventually became apparent that objections to the hybrid Morin model fell into three distinct categories. Some program designers felt that the refinements and unique features of their specific interventions might be misrepresented if translated into the terminology adopted by Morin. Others were bothered by the suggestion—never made by Morin himself—that linear progress from one level or belief to another was expected or required. Finally, one outspoken exception-taker assumed—without realizing that Morin himself had drawn heavily from a very successful program to reduce cholesterol intake and overall risk for hypertension among Black men in the Baltimore area—that a model used to shape prevention support for gay White men could not possibly have any relevance to programs developed for other population groups.

COORDINATING THE ELEMENTS

Very early in the epidemic, the Department of Public Health assumed responsibility for coordinating the overall prevention effort in San Francisco. The Department allocated the initial funding for the prevention effort to gay-identifying organizations committed to preventing the further spread of a deadly disease, which in 1982 seemed to affect homosexual and bisexual men almost exclusively. Later, injection drug users were also identified as a high-risk group, although early in the epidemic there was almost complete overlap of these two groups.[4]

From the beginning, Department staff were acutely aware that the prevention effort was attempting to change the behavior of people who historically had been oppressed and were distrustful of government. Early population-based surveys confirmed credibility problems with public officials among gay men and needle users. The same problem emerged as the risk of ethnic communities for HIV became more apparent. As a result, the centerpiece of DPH's response in each case has been to engage community-based organizations closely identified with these population groups to spearhead prevention efforts.

The first Department contract with a community-based organization focused on HIV prevention was funded in December 1982 and capped at $48,200. Within six months, the AIDS Office had been established by the director of health to coordinate efforts and administer all AIDS-specific contracts; within fifteen months, there were four more AIDS education and prevention contractors, and *in toto*, their city-funded budgets were almost ten times the 1982 contract amount. Five years later, in 1989, there were 32 community-based organizations contracting with DPH offices for HIV prevention services. In addition, there was a wide range of AIDS-specific prevention efforts being managed directly by eight administrative subdivisions of the Department itself (e.g., by the city's STD clinic, maternal and child health clinics). By 1989 government funding for all prevention programs totaled almost $8 million, and 47 percent of the total was associated with programs serving ethnic communities.

Between 1982 and 1989, a major consideration in the designation of government funds to HIV prevention services was to support programs for which there was sufficient aggregate funding available (from any combination of sources) to mount a meaningful effort. This was often referred to as the *critical mass*. A corollary concern was to avoid fragmenting prevention work among a large number of underfunded or precariously funded entities whose energies would subsequently be focused on securing more funds rather than on the prevention effort itself. The potential for sustaining a particular effort over time was a third major concern shaping decisions about funding specific programs.

It became the AIDS Office's responsibility to ensure that the aggregate government funding for each participating community-based organization or subdivision of the Department was stable and expanded only when there was a reasonable prospect of maintaining the expanded program. Between 1982 and 1989, the AIDS Office was able to assure all providers of a stable and often expanding base, even in years when categorical federal or state support for particular efforts was arbitrarily cut back. Overall, federal and state funding for HIV programs increased steadily during this period, but local government funds were often shifted from one program area to another, as needed, to counterbalance shifts in support from other sources for particular types of programs.*

Having a single local entity (the AIDS Office within the Department of Public Health) consistently assume the central role in channeling funding for the overall HIV prevention effort to local providers undoubtedly resulted in greater total funding, particularly federal funding, for San Francisco's programs. Applications for such funding became cooperative ventures and were frequently recognized and rewarded for the collaboration.

In keeping with the theme of engaging the communities and members of subcultures most heavily impacted by the HIV epidemic as partners in the process, the Department sought to have these communities and interests well represented on the staff of its offices charged with responding to the epidemic. From the start, openly gay men and lesbians at DPH were assigned key roles in coordinating the city's response to AIDS. As the need to work more closely with ethnic communities became apparent, the ethnic diversity of the staffs of departmental offices working with AIDS also was expanded.

Identifying Appropriate Providers

Prevention program designers speak of "providers" delivering "messages" to target "audiences" using one or more of the "approaches" described. This description tends to make the process sound very managed, hierarchical and prescriptive. For the most part, however, San Francisco programs have involved the people and communities whose understanding and behavior is expected to change as partners in the process. It has been a given that the values and norms of both individuals and communities must be respected

---

* Federal and state appropriations for home-based health care and related support services have been far more erratic than appropriations for prevention programs. By 1989 the vast majority of the less restricted funds from local government had to be committed to out-of-hospital care and support.

and that their social networks must be fully engaged if behavior changes are to be adopted and maintained.

The community-based organizations involved in the early years of the epidemic were those that presented themselves to the Department as willing and able to do the job. In identifying providers to receive government funding for frontline risk-reduction services (whether community-based organizations or subdivisions within DPH itself), the Department accepted the premise that providers should be evaluated by the following criteria: (a) their credibility among the audiences targeted; (b) their ability to articulate a program plan and to link it to specific information available about the knowledge, attitudes, beliefs and behaviors of those targeted; (c) their willingness and ability to adjust a program plan if new information about knowledge, attitudes, beliefs and behaviors of those targeted warrants such adjustment; and (d) their willingness and ability to account for their activities and the use of funds received in a way that permits a reasonable assessment of cost and impact.

Community-based providers have been encouraged to augment government funding with contributions from the private sector in the form of cash donations as well as in-kind support. Over the years, it has been shown that it is in the provider's own interest to establish cash reserves to meet cash flow requirements, which contracts based on reimbursement for actual costs incurred do not provide. It has also become apparent that the fundraising process itself substantially increases awareness of the need for prevention and supports behavior change in targeted communities.

Local government funding of gay-identifying organizations began in December 1982, when 134 cases of AIDS had been reported in San Francisco, 97 percent of which were among homosexual or bisexual men. AIDS-specific funding for community-based organizations working with substance abusers began in March 1985, by which time 15 percent of the 1,006 cases of AIDS reported to date were among injection drug users; homosexual and bisexual men comprised 95 percent of these injection drug users. Some of these community-based organizations working with injection drug users were also identified with specific ethnic communities. In July 1986 direct funding for more general AIDS outreach to ethnic communities was provided by the State of California directly to two community-based organizations in San Francisco. This was at a time when 14 percent of the 2,531 cases of AIDS reported to date were from ethnic groups. At the time, homosexual and bisexual men, many of them gay-identified, comprised nearly 90 percent of these ethnic minority AIDS cases.[5]

When audiences have been defined by the location in which they are available to be educated, San Francisco's program planners have relied largely on offices and agencies traditionally responsible for services in those locations. The activities of these agencies also provide a mix of general awareness and risk reduction support. For example, DPH's Forensic Services has been responsible for AIDS education for jail/detention facility staff as well as for inmates and detainees. The San Francisco Unified School District, working with staff of DPH's Community Public Health Services, has focused on school staff development regarding AIDS, as well as on programs targeting youth in school. City Clinic (San Francisco's public clinic for sexually transmitted diseases) and other government supported health centers have assumed responsibility for HIV education and prevention programs for patients and individuals targeted in their outreach services.

Which Approaches? Which Messages?

With different degrees of commitment and success, San Francisco's HIV education and prevention programs follow two general principles. The first has been that all messages should be consistent with the latest developments in epidemiological and medical knowledge about HIV and its transmission. The second has been that messages should be conveyed through a medium (print, pictures, oral/aural), in language (visual, verbal) and in a setting that the targeted audience will be able to understand, will find appropriate and to which it will respond. The general approach or delivery mechanism and the "spin" of particular messages, however, may vary dramatically.

The factors that determine which general approaches and specific messages are used include: (1) who is targeted; (2) what the audience already knows and believes; (3) what exposure the audience has already had; (4) what literacy/education levels can be assumed;

(5) which media are to be used; (6) what levels of formality and intimacy the audience will respond to; (7) who is delivering the message; (8) what factors contributing to health-related attitudes and/or barriers to behavior change are being addressed; (9) what the particular goal of the educational intervention is; and (10) what resources are available. Each program component is expected to seek answers to these questions from a variety of sources. The major sources of information are discussed below.

• *Providers' knowledge of their constituents:* San Francisco's overall prevention program has relied heavily on the insights of frontline providers to design specific interventions for the audiences for which they have assumed responsibility. In the early years, AIDS Office staff working with community-based providers relied on the premise that it was the job of the community-based organization contractors to understand the needs of their respective constituencies and to interpret for the AIDS Office the programmatic implications of surveys and seroprevalence data. For the AIDS Office, the primary concern was that contractors had a clear and well-articulated rationale for doing what they had done and planned to do.

• *Focus groups and field testing mechanisms*: The Department's AIDS Office has expected frontline providers, as a matter of practice, to utilize focus groups and other qualitative assessments to refine the implications of population-based surveys as well as to preview draft materials and strategies. By 1985 contracts with the AIDS Office specifically limited AIDS Office staff review of strategies and materials to consideration of (a) statements of medical fact made or implied and (b) the process by which representatives of populations targeted were engaged in the development of strategies and materials.

The process by which representatives were selected for such groups has been pivotal. Materials developed for injection drug users out of treatment, for example, had to be reviewed by one or more focus groups of injection drug users out of treatment. Recovering injection drug users or staff members of treatment programs could participate in the process and offer their insights, but at some point the review had to involve the actual audience concerned.

• *Data from cohort studies:* Several prospective studies of the epidemiology of HIV infection have been undertaken in San Francisco. Planners of prevention programs have been encouraged to use data on knowledge, attitudes, beliefs and behaviors gathered from participants in the cohorts being followed in these studies. Most of these cohort studies also provide information about the HIV antibody status of their participants and patterns of seroconversion.

• *Data from community surveys*: San Francisco has pioneered the use of periodic population-based surveys of knowledge, attitudes, beliefs and behaviors to help shape and assess its prevention efforts. Some have been telephone surveys and others, door-to-door surveys. The first such survey was undertaken in 1984 among self-identified gay and bisexual men of all ethnicities. Since then, multiple surveys have been conducted of this population, as well as of heterosexuals with multiple or high-risk partners of all ethnicities and the Black and Hispanic communities (low- as well as high-risk individuals). Baseline surveys of the Chinese, Japanese, Filipino, Korean and Southeast Asian communities also were undertaken in 1988 and 1989.

In 1989 the Department of Public Health also contracted for a special survey of ethnic homosexual and bisexual men with participants recruited through ethnic gay organizations, bars, social clubs and their social networks. This was done because the population-based surveys did not yield large enough samples of homosexual and bisexual men from ethnic communities to assess the behavior changes and needs of these particular high-risk groups.

The purpose of these surveys, over time, is to: (a) evaluate AIDS knowledge, attitudes, beliefs and behavior changes in high-risk and ethnic populations in San Francisco; (b) evaluate health education/ risk reduction programs; (c) assess behavioral changes over time that might affect trends of HIV infection; and (d) enable prevention and education programs to better target interventions and maximize resources.

LIMITING THE PREVENTION AGENDA

San Francisco has been relatively successful in keeping its programs well focused on prevention efforts that constructively support the development of behaviors that reduce the risk of transmission of HIV. In working with gay and bisexual men, for example, San Francisco's programs have made no attempt to discourage participants from living their lives fully as gay-identifying or bisexual men. Rather, these programs have limited their expectations of change to the specific behaviors that put participants at risk of HIV infection.

Where substance abuse may be a factor in transmission, the goals of San Francisco's programs may be best described as incremental and pragmatic. The initial goal has been to end the sharing of contaminated needles and the unsafe sexual activity associated with substance use, even though the larger goal has been to end the substance use that encourages needle sharing and unsafe sexual activity. It has also been apparent from the beginning that the transmission of HIV was not likely to be controlled if HIV prevention efforts were focused on this larger goal.

EDUCATING THE GENERAL PUBLIC

San Francisco's overall HIV prevention effort also has rested on the tenet that, to be effective, the overall program must establish a general environment in which interventions targeted to those specifically at risk are understood as constructive by all segments of the community. This requires outreach and education to the general public, which directly and indirectly supports outreach to specific high-risk groups.

Education of the general public must include efforts to persuade all segments of the population—those at high risk and those who are not—that everyone has a role in risk reduction. Broad goals of outreach to the public include: (a) fostering general awareness about the transmission of HIV and how individuals can protect themselves and others from infection; (b) fostering general awareness among the HIV-infected, asymptomatic population about the importance of health-promoting behaviors and the availability of sound medical options, including early intervention with drug treatments; (c) demystifying HIV and as a result, reducing fear and hysteria about casual transmission; and (d) fostering an understanding of the dimensions of the problem, its complexity and the potential costs (in terms of lives and dollars), so support for constructive and cost-effective services will be forthcoming.

It is equally important that education of the general public about AIDS confronts prejudices associated with the groups most directly affected by HIV, prejudices that were deep seated long before the onset of the AIDS epidemic. Nationally *and* locally, the vast majority of those who have developed AIDS are members of behavioral minorities (homosexual/bisexual men and injection drug users). Of the 7,686 AIDS cases reported in San Francisco between 1981 and December 1989, 97.5 percent are in these categories.[6]

SUMMARY

This chapter identifies three dimensions used in the descriptive framework adopted for San Francisco's overall prevention model: audiences, approaches and messages. It explains how organizations with roots in the communities and subcultures most highly impacted by the epidemic have been engaged by the local department of health and have played a central role in the development and implementation of prevention programs that have emerged. The next chapter examines several critical junctures at which the cooperative venture undertaken by the Department of Public Health and community-based organizations has been severely tested.

San Francisco's Prevention Partnership: Issues and Challenges

Jeffery W. Amory

INTRODUCTION

One recurring theme has dominated San Francisco's experience with HIV prevention: namely, the strength of the partnership forged between public health officials and organizations and individuals with roots in the communities and subcultures most heavily affected by the epidemic.

The idea of partnerships was first introduced in 1982 when the Department of Public Health (DPH) contracted with an organization then known as the Kaposi's Sarcoma Research and Education Foundation to spearhead an effort to educate the city's gay community about a disease that at the time was widely referred to as "the gay plague." The organization, which later changed its name to the San Francisco AIDS Foundation, had emerged as a grass-roots effort within the gay community and reflected a growing recognition among gay people that the disease was "our problem." Within 15 months, the Department had contracts with four other prevention providers closely identified with San Francisco's gay community; by 1984 the pattern of enlisting partnerships with community-based organizations was well established.

The Department's early contracting with gay-identifying organizations stemmed from the recognition that the individuals most seriously affected by the HIV epidemic had a long history of rejection by American society and that this sense of alienation persisted for many gay men, even in San Francisco. More to the point, many gay men and lesbians were openly skeptical about the city's concern for their welfare.* It was apparent that a prevention effort undertaken directly by DPH would encounter much more resistance from the targeted population than one undertaken by organizations with strong roots in the community itself. Community-based organizations, it was also believed, would be able to draw strength and cohesion from the sense of shared alienation and discrimination. A few years later, when ethnic communities were recognized as populations needing more carefully targeted HIV prevention efforts, it was relatively easy for the Department to expand on this concept.

From the beginning, therefore, San Francisco's overall HIV prevention effort took on many of the characteristics of a cooperative venture between the Department of Public Health and private, not-for-profit organizations with roots in the communities most heavily affected. In this effort, community or subculture identity and group ownership of the problem have been the key variables in the city's prevention effort. Public health "experts" have served as much as partners to the communities involved as they have as direct prevention program providers.

San Francisco's commitment to this community-based approach has been tested at several junctures over the years. The "bathhouse controversy," which dominated headlines and discussions of HIV

---

* This skepticism had recently been reinforced by the official response to the assassination of Harvey Milk, San Francisco's first gay-identified member of the Board of Supervisors, and Mayor George Moscone, his political ally. In the 1979 verdict that many regarded as reflective of the local establishment's attitude toward the gay community, the man who had confessed to shooting Milk and Moscone was found guilty only of manslaughter, which carried a maximum sentence of less than eight years and provided prospects of parole within five.

prevention in 1984, was the first serious test of San Francisco's commitment to this approach. The second test came when the HIV antibody test was licensed by the Food and Drug Administration (FDA) in 1985, and political pressure began to mount outside of the city, with ramifications for the city, to institute widespread HIV antibody testing, with the reporting of names of those who tested positive. The third juncture came in 1986 when conflicts developed over which community-based organizations would best serve the growing needs for HIV prevention of San Francisco's ethnic communities. The fourth critical period is still in progress and results from policies and procedures adopted by DPH that have created the perception by many that community-based contractors have been demoted from their status as full partners in the city's overall prevention effort.

THE BATHHOUSE CONTROVERSY

Between March and September 1984, when the debate about closing the city's bathhouses was at its peak in San Francisco, HIV prevention was still regarded primarily as a concern of the gay community. This controversy tested the commitment of government and the public health establishment in San Francisco to work cooperatively with gay community institutions in combating AIDS.

During the 1970s, bathhouses had played an important role in the liberation of the gay community. By the early 1980s, the bathhouses, although actually used by a small minority of gay and bisexual men, had become well established in gay culture as places where men could meet and have sex in environments that were relatively well sheltered from external intrusions. Because of the presumed role that larger numbers of sexual partners had in the transmission of HIV infection (an activity that bathhouses allowed and some claim, encouraged), pressure began building on San Francisco's Director of Health, Dr. Mervyn Silverman, to intervene and close the bathhouses. By the end of June 1983, more than two hundred cases of AIDS had been reported in San Francisco, and the city had averaged 18 new cases per month during the first six months of that year. These were alarming statistics. The pressure to close the bathhouses was evident in comments made by some political leaders (both straight and gay, but most notably by then-Mayor Dianne Feinstein), by some health care professionals (many of them gay) who were treating people with AIDS, as well as in newspaper editorials and in sometimes slanted reports that appeared in the city's major newspapers.

The alarm and the pressure notwithstanding, several factors seemed to mitigate against this kind of intervention by the county's health officer. Many of those staffing the recently established HIV prevention programs argued that bathhouses provided excellent locations for aggressive promotion of HIV prevention among sexually active gay men, especially those who did not readily identify themselves as part of the gay community. Mentioned more than once in the debate was the danger to wives who could perhaps become infected through their bisexual husbands who had gone to the bathhouses to have sex with anonymous male partners. These locations, the argument went, could serve as places for the distribution of literature and for forums and special events targeted to such hard-to-reach audiences. If the bathhouses were closed, such activity would move to parks and alleys, where the men who most needed to be educated would be less accessible to prevention messages.

The situation was further complicated by the fact that bathhouses were, at the time, licensed by the police department. Any public hearings regarding their closure would undoubtedly have raised more dramatically the specter of police harassment of gay men for their sexuality, which would have undermined the Department's main strategy of working cooperatively with the gay community to promote HIV risk reduction. Furthermore, while it was common knowledge that sexual activity took place at bathhouses and sex clubs, there were no hard data available about the incidence of specific acts that put patrons at high risk for infection. Such data would be needed to support the health officer's order to close.

Late in March 1984, a longtime gay activist who had written repeatedly to the director of health and the board of supervisors formally announced that he was seeking a ballot measure to ban sex in San Francisco bathhouses.* This action precipitated a firestorm of

---

*By this time, the term "bathhouses" was commonly used to encompass all business locations in which sex between men took place.

debate within San Francisco's gay community itself and put much more direct pressure on Silverman, the director of health, to intervene. The rhetoric was passionate and the divisions ran deep. All the arguments cited earlier were repeated. The one new argument put forward was that the health officer should close all the city's bathhouses, sex clubs and gay-oriented adult video- and bookstores to preempt the ballot initiative. It was feared that a vote to close the bathhouses would be interpreted as a major setback for gay rights in the city.

After almost two weeks of marathon meetings with gay community groups, physicians, epidemiologists, the press and city attorneys, Silverman announced he wanted to close the bathhouses because of their contribution to the transmission of HIV. To this end, he formally requested that licensing and regulatory authority for bathhouses be transferred from the police department to the health department. Official responses from the police department, the mayor and the board of supervisors were postponed for a variety of reasons, and the transfer of authority never occurred. Within two months, however, Silverman concluded a second round of meetings on the issue and announced that he was closing the bathhouses under the admittedly more tenuous authority he already had as health officer. By this time, he also had reports by private investigators in hand that detailed an incidence of high-risk sexual behavior that seemed to him sufficient to justify his intervening in this manner.

Subsequently, a restraining order was requested by a group of bathhouse owners and issued by a superior court judge, and the health officer's discretionary authority was limited to overseeing the implementation of certain structural changes (e.g., doors to private rooms had to be cut two feet from the floor) and monitoring patron behavior. The general thrust of the court's order was to keep the businesses open but at the same time, to restrict behavior and to use the sites as forums for promoting HIV risk reduction.

Significance of the Bathhouse Controversy

The bathhouse controversy is significant in the history of San Francisco's response to the HIV epidemic because it provided a critical test of the Department of Public Health's commitment to the principles underlying the overall prevention effort to date. On the whole, DPH's commitment to these principles remained intact. Silverman, in particular, maintained his personal commitment to working with the gay community as partners in the decision-making process. Every group he met with to discuss his options included a significant proportion (in most cases a majority) of gay men and lesbians among the medical professionals, political activists and other advice givers. His major problem was that the gay community itself was deeply divided on the issue and he had to choose sides.

Subsequent Developments

In the months that followed the attempt to close the bathhouses, people involved in the controversy seemed to move on to other issues. Most of the bathhouses and many sex clubs eventually went out of business for lack of business. The collaboration between public health officials and the gay-identifying organizations working on HIV prevention in the community was, in the long run, not seriously harmed by the controversy. Subsequently, many took the position that the controversy itself made an important contribution to the diffusion of information among gay and bisexual men regarding risk reduction.

Since 1987 several private clubs have emerged in the city at which gay men meet for sex. Their existence is noted periodically in the press and their activities are monitored, but the controversy that surrounded the initial closing of the bathhouses has not been rekindled.

THE HIV ANTIBODY TEST

The bathhouse controversy played itself out, by and large, as a controversy among individuals and factions within San Francisco. Most of the contributors to this discussion were themselves gay. In sharp contrast, the controversy over the appropriate role of HIV antibody testing in HIV prevention was cast between "outsiders" (non-San Franciscans), on one hand, who were advocating mandatory testing and registering the names of people who tested positive, and concerned individuals and factions within the city, both straight and gay, on the other, who reflected a remarkable degree of consensus in their conviction that such an approach would be counterproductive to prevention efforts. At the time, the threat of discrimination against people who tested HIV-positive seemed to concerned San Franciscans sufficient to ensure that such a strategy would put those at high risk at odds with the health care delivery system. As a result, these individuals would be driven away from legitimate prevention programs and clinical services.

In many states, confidential registries of persons infected with particular sexually transmitted diseases (STDs), such as syphilis and hepatitis, are maintained by state or local officials. With such STDs, health care providers test and treat index cases and report their names to the registry. Public health officials follow up by notifying the sexual partners of those initially screened. The partners are then tested and treated if treatment is indicated. The names of the partners who test positive are also reported to the registry. If the system works as intended, the pattern is repeated with all subsequent partners of each person who tests positive until the treatments and notifications catch up with the infection. Most public health officials consider this the standard procedure for controlling the spread of STDs.

While HIV is sexually transmitted, it is different in some crucial ways from other infections that public health officials attempt to control by reporting names, notifying partners and treating the infection. For example, in contrast to the relatively short period between infection and the development of symptoms with other reportable STDs, the incubation period for HIV is very long (more than ten years in many cases). Even antibodies to HIV are typically not detectable until three months and, in rare cases, as much as three years after infection.[1] In addition, there is no known cure for HIV disease. Even with recent medical developments, the most people infected with HIV can reasonably expect from clinical interventions is a delay in onset of symptoms and an average life expectancy after a diagnosis of clinical AIDS that has increased from 14 months to 21 months.[2] To most San Franciscans working to end the epidemic, these differences between HIV infection and other sexually transmitted diseases were sufficient to warrant a waiver of standard procedures.

In early 1985, the Food and Drug Administration licensed a relatively inexpensive assay, or test, for the presence of HIV antibodies, whose acronym is ELISA. ELISA is highly sensitive and specific for antibodies to HIV. Its licensing meant that a testing mechanism for standard STD control procedure was now available for HIV as well. Since the test has been licensed, there has been considerable and highly politicized pressure from some politicians and public health officials outside of San Francisco to implement mandatory testing, registry of names and partner notification procedures for HIV-affected populations. Concurrently, there has been strong resistance to such a strategy from others. In California the debate has been particularly heated. Between 1986 and 1988, proposals for mandatory testing and state-managed registries for those who test positive were twice put before the voters in the form of ballot initiatives and defeated.

Mandatory Testing and Reporting

Much of the political and financial support for mandatory testing and reporting the names of people who test positive has come from organizations whose rhetoric has been laced with presumptions about the "immorality" of homosexual behavior, the equation of all homosexual behavior with high risk for HIV infection and the corollary that there are "guilty" sufferers and "innocent" victims of HIV infection. The anti-gay shadow that has accompanied much of the discussion reflects the fact that AIDS has, from the beginning, had its greatest impact on this stigmatized minority, whose homosexuality is presumed by some to be reprehensible and perhaps even the "cause" of their illness. Matters have been further complicated because the next highest incidence of AIDS is among injection drug users, and nationally, although not in San Francisco, the incidence of reported AIDS cases is disproportionately high among ethnic minorities, all stigmatized or marginalized populations.

In short, the HIV epidemic has exacerbated long-standing problems of prejudice and bias. The potential for using HIV test results to foster discrimination has been obvious to all parties in the debate;

the more vocal advocates of mandatory testing have made it clear they think that such discrimination is appropriate.

In San Francisco, however, both the political and public health establishments were quick to recognize the extent to which the full cooperation of people infected and at risk is important in controlling the spread of HIV and the extent to which the perceived threat of discrimination would discourage vital cooperation. From the beginning, these forces in San Francisco have been virtually unanimous in their opposition to mandatory testing and to reporting the names of those who test positive, except where blood donations were concerned.

Voluntary Testing and Counseling Programs

Notwithstanding the general opposition to mandatory testing and reporting the names of those who test positive, voluntary testing and related counseling have played a large and important role in San Francisco's overall HIV prevention effort.*

In July 1985, the Department of Public Health initiated a program of HIV antibody testing at anonymous test sites (ATS) throughout the city. Since its inception, the ATS program has been promoted as a prevention education and counseling program that uses test results as a catalyst for stimulating or reinforcing new patterns of low-risk behavior. The basic safeguards of this anonymous testing are, first, no personal identifying information on program participants is sought or recorded, and second, staff of the testing program have no job-related responsibilities outside the ATS program that are likely to put them in contact with those tested. The purpose of the second safeguard is to provide reasonable assurances that staff members will not be able to identify a person tested because of knowledge gained from other job-related interactions.

These programs in San Francisco have probably tested more people per capita than any other local public health jurisdiction in the coun-

---

* It has been assumed that, for some, knowledge of their antibody status would play a critical role in persuading them to initiate or maintain necessary behavior changes. However, there was and continues to be no conclusive evidence to support the hypothesis that knowledge of one's antibody status consistently plays a role in persuading one to initiate or maintain behavior changes.

try.* However, great care has been taken in these programs to ensure that all components work with participants as partners in combating the transmission of HIV and that none of them compromise the civil rights of people who are tested. Participants in these programs are carefully counseled in pre- and post-test sessions.

Testing Donated Blood

While most HIV antibody testing services were developed slowly, to insure that all implications were weighed and all consequences considered, the use of the antibody test to screen blood donations was not delayed. The need for and appropriateness of using the antibody test to screen blood donations has never been seriously contested since ELISA became available in 1985.

Before ELISA was licensed by the FDA, people receiving blood transfusions were at risk for HIV. At the time, it was unclear how high the risk was. Pre-1985 efforts to reduce this risk focused on discouraging the donation of blood by people in known high-risk groups, specifically gay/bisexual men and injection drug users. Since the test was licensed and its use in screening blood donations became mandatory, further transmission through transfusions has been effectively controlled by screening all blood used in transfusions. A small risk remains, nevertheless, because of the three month window it typically takes to develop antibodies to HIV.

Also since 1985, heat treatment of all coagulation factor concentrates has effectively controlled further spread of HIV to hemophiliacs through their use of blood products.

Partner Notification

In San Francisco, partner notification, sometimes called "contact tracing," has been limited to heterosexual partners of persons diagnosed with AIDS, recipients of blood donated by people later diagnosed with AIDS, and partners of persons who are known by their physician to be HIV antibody positive *and* who request their

---

* Between March 1985 and October 1989, 51,363 tests were performed at San Francisco's anonymous test sites alone. Factoring in tests done as part of routine clinical screening in both public and private settings (21,614) and making allowances for multiple tests for some individuals, the DPH AIDS Office estimates that 84 per 1,000 population have been tested.[3]

physician to assist them in notifying their partners. The first two reflect local public health policy; the last is required by state law. No community-based organizations have been involved in this aspect of prevention work in San Francisco.

An analysis of the effectiveness and cost of the contact tracing program for heterosexual partners of persons diagnosed with AIDS was made by the Department of Public Health AIDS Office in 1987.[4] The study revealed that fewer than 16 percent of the first generation of sexual partners could be contacted. Largely because of the long incubation period of HIV, the vast majority of partners were lost to followup. In addition, the cost totaled approximately $400 per partner reached and tested. It was judged that the inefficiency of contact tracing and the resulting cost would be significantly greater in population groups where there was a high incidence of HIV infection, such as gay men or injection drug users. This inefficiency and high cost, coupled with the strategic arguments against widespread use of partner notification in the overall prevention effort, have ensured a very minor and restricted role for contact tracing in the overall effort. Since contact tracing is a natural extension of a strategy of testing and reporting, whatever controversy has touched on contact tracing in San Francisco has highlighted questions about the larger issues of testing and reporting.

Subsequent Developments

Throughout 1987, as medical research began to suggest that early clinical interventions had some efficacy for those who are HIV-positive but asymptomatic, HIV antibody testing and related counseling programs were established in clinical health care settings. The testing in these instances has been confidential rather than anonymous. Confidential test results are associated with patients' names, albeit in a separate record, access to which is restricted by California state law and further by local administrative policy. In addition, fully informed consent is required from those tested. At these clinic sites, HIV testing is done in the context of a more general medical examination, and it constitutes screening in the usual sense.

By 1989 DPH and the community-based organizations involved in the anonymous testing program were recommending that people who felt themselves to be at risk be tested and counseled about both preventing HIV transmission and about the emerging protocols for early clinical intervention for those who test positive, including the use of AZT and aerosolized pentamidine. The emphasis on voluntary testing and the opposition to reporting the names of those who test positive has never been abandoned, however.

OUTREACH TO ETHNIC COMMUNITIES

In 1986, a number of conflicting perceptions and expectations among advocacy and provider groups in San Francisco began to receive public attention. For the most part, these conflicts were expressed as differences over which providers were entitled to claim which audiences, how funding levels for outreach to particular audiences should be established and how services should be described. Advocacy groups representing ethnic minority interests, for example, stated that HIV prevention efforts targeting ethnic minority populations should be operated only by community-based providers identified with these communities. Others initially took the position that ethnic minority subsets of their target populations (gay men, for example, or substance abusers or female clients of family planning services) could be and were being well served by organizations operating under broader missions.

Much of the discussion of these issues was driven by evidence that ethnic communities were disproportionately represented among reported AIDS cases nationally. Although this disproportionate impact had not materialized in San Francisco, the national figures made it clear that more aggressive and well-targeted prevention efforts needed to be focused on these communities. At the same time, there were data indicating that the rate of new HIV infections among ethnic populations in San Francisco was rising, which added to the urgency of the situation.

Initial Response
Without rejecting the position that some individuals from ethnic communities were already being well served by umbrella-styled

programs, the Department recognized that more had to be done for the Black, Hispanic, Asian/Pacific Islander and Native American communities. In 1986, several specific steps were taken to underscore this awareness. First, representatives of advocacy and provider groups associated with ethnic community interests were incorporated into a network of formal advisory bodies to the new Director of Health, Dr. David Werdegar.

Second, specific community-based organizations identified by these ethnic community advisory groups were recognized as having unique access to the target communities and were engaged as HIV education and prevention providers. Funding for these new programs was secured and expanded each year for several years. In keeping with the earlier policy of underwriting only programs for which a critical mass of funding was available, one primary contractor was identified for each of four community groups (Black, Latino, Asian/ Pacific Islander and Native American). Contracts with all-minority providers who presented themselves as multicultural augmented these services.

Third, the Department requested more refined demographic breakdowns of audiences reached by every HIV prevention provider, so a clearer picture of the overall impact of HIV prevention efforts on ethnic minority audiences could be attained.

In 1986-87, there was $3.6 million in government funding for HIV education and prevention support programs in San Francisco. Of this total, $1.4 million or 38 percent was identified as having an impact on ethnic populations. Forty-one percent or $570,000 of the minority impact funding went to community-based organizations working exclusively with specific ethnic communities. The balance, $820,000, was associated with efforts targeted to populations first defined by characteristics other than their ethnicity—populations defined by gender, for example, sexual orientation or the location or setting where the education takes place (e.g., in school, jail, the workplace)—but a portion of whose audiences were also from ethnic communities.[5]

By 1988-89, government funding for HIV education and prevention support programs in San Francisco had grown to $7.9 million. Of this total, 47 percent or $3.5 million was associated with impact on ethnic communities. Forty-five percent of the $3.5 million, $1.7 million, was assigned to community-based organizations working exclusively with ethnic communities.[6]

Subsequent Developments

Anecdotal feedback has been mixed regarding the success of attempts since 1986 to engage fully the community identity of Blacks, Hispanics, Asians/Pacific Islanders and Native Americans in HIV prevention. For example, although men who have sex with other men (but who may not identify themselves as gay or bisexual) are clearly the individuals at highest risk for HIV in San Francisco's ethnic communities,[7] most HIV prevention programs identified with these communities have experienced difficulty with outreach to this segment of their constituency, difficulty that is related primarily to cultural taboos about homosexual behavior.

Some programs also have found certain aspects of their community identity to be much less cohesive than the four-group model adopted by the Department. The Asian AIDS Project, for example, has had special challenges stemming from the fact that the Asian/ Pacific Islander community in San Francisco is made up of more than 30 distinct language and cultural groups.

The basic policy question raised by these observations is: How far is it reasonable and necessary to carry a commitment to working with community identity in developing HIV prevention programs? Put another way, the question would be: At what point does the division of limited funding among more community-based organizations (each representing a more discretely defined constituency) become counterproductive because it results in organizations so underfunded that their energies are focused on securing funds rather than on the prevention effort itself?

In terms of the specific issue of funding HIV prevention programs in San Francisco's ethnic communities, the question might be: Is it necessary and feasible to fund separate prevention providers for each minority community-at-large, other providers for the subcultures in each community of men who have sex with other men and still other providers who claim to accommodate many of these men because of their self-identification as gay? Another might be: Should the various Asian/Pacific Islander communities, who together account for more than 25 percent of the population but fewer than 2 percent of the reported AIDS cases, each have a separate program?

There has been some movement on the part of the AIDS Office and its contractors in the direction of a clearer focus on the needs of men of color who have sex with other men. Whether this will result in direct funding for new provider organizations or greater emphasis in established organizations on prevention support for these men remains to be determined.

CHALLENGES TO THE PARTNERSHIP

Over time the commitment of the Department of Public Health and contracting community-based organizations to working as full partners in the fight against AIDS has, perhaps inevitably, diminished. Several factors have contributed to this development. The effect on the communities targeted by their programs has not yet been assessed.

The Impact of Growth

The first factor stems from the dramatic growth in the number of community-based organizations involved in the HIV prevention effort, as well as from the expansion of the bureaucracies at DPH and at cooperating community-based organizations. The overall sense of mission that characterized the early partnerships has been watered down considerably by the increase in the number of players.

This effect has been compounded by the fact that many of the newer contractors for AIDS prevention services have been organizations with a history of contracting with the Department for the provision of other kinds of services, such as mental health and substance abuse treatment. This previous contracting experience, which often had adversarial overtones, sometimes created obstacles to the new relationships the Department was trying to establish with these organizations. In addition, new staff at the AIDS Office sometimes arrived on the job with expectations of a more "junior partner" role for contractors.

Censorship of Materials

The second factor can be traced to the distinct break that newly appointed Department staff made in 1987-8 with the tradition of a very restricted AIDS Office role in the review of materials developed by contracting community-based organizations.

In the early years of the partnership and in language incorporated into all contracts between community-based organizations and the AIDS Office, AIDS Office review of materials and strategies was strictly limited to consideration of statements of medical fact made or implied and the process by which representatives of populations targeted were engaged in program development. As federal and state funding became more available to support HIV prevention programs, further restrictions began to be imposed by federal and state agencies on the language and approaches their funding could be used to support.

In 1986 the California Department of Health Services (DHS) began requiring that all materials to be produced or distributed using state funds be submitted to their Office of AIDS for review and approval. DHS specifically prohibited "slang," making it clear that this meant the kind of language most individuals at risk would use in normal, everyday conversation. A few months later, the federal Centers for Disease Control required all recipients of their funds to establish a local review panel "to consider the bounds of explicitness believed needed to communicate an effective message to those for whom it is intended." In October 1987, the panel's enforcement mandate was expanded by the Helms amendment, named after conservative Senator Jesse Helms (R-N.C.). The amendment prohibited programs receiving federal funding for HIV prevention from using "materials and activities that promote or encourage, directly, homosexual sexual activities."

As the designated recipient of most of the state and federal funding subject to this censorship, the AIDS Office stood between the community-based organizations developing materials and approaches and the federal and state agency censors. The AIDS Office and its contractors agreed that these restrictions were onerous and fundamentally inconsistent with the principles on which programs had been based. As a practical matter, however, the major difficulty was posed by the state's bureaucratically managed procedures. San Francisco has not experienced problems with federal censorship because the federally approved local review panel has been disinclined to let abstract notions of propriety interfere with aggressive and meaningful prevention efforts. The potential for restrictions by state reviewers was itself minimized by ensuring, insofar as possible, that no program was completely dependent on state funding; most programs were provided other resources to underwrite costs the state government would be unlikely to approve.

It is particularly ironic that it was DPH's handling of its own local review requirements that has risked undermining the Department and community-based organization partnership. Between 1987 and 1989, interventions by senior DPH staff in the production of materials developed by community-based organizations increased dramatically. In many cases, the reasons for these interventions had nothing to do either with statements of medical fact or with the process by which representatives of populations targeted were engaged in the development of materials—the criteria for DPH in-house review spelled out in contracts. Many community-based organizations complained about the incursions into "their turf" as well as the time that it took to get materials and plans reviewed.

The principle of a partnership that values equally the contributions of both the public health establishment and community-based organizations was challenged by such interventions. These interventions were curtailed in 1989, but their legacy continues to shadow some of the dialogue between the AIDS Office and community-based organizations.

Changes in Contracting Policies

In most local public health jurisdictions, the participation of community-based organizations in HIV prevention program delivery is sought through competitive bidding undertaken after local, state or federal funding is secured by the department of health. In such situations, the status of contracting community-based organizations is clearly subservient to the local government agency managing the funding.

Prior to 1989, the AIDS Office, with the approval of the Health

Commission, issued requests for competitive bids (often referred to as Requests For Proposals, or RFPs) *only* in situations where there was obviously more than one viable and interested candidate. In addition, once a contractor was established for a particular array of services, the contractor was generally incorporated into the AIDS Office's own applications for funding as a co-applicant. All such applications were routinely reviewed and approved by the Health Commission, the policymaking body governing the Department. State and federal funding offices had made it clear that such applications were rated higher if they reflected full participation by community-based organizations with a track record in the area of service being funded.

In 1989, however, the Health Commission reversed this position and required that all contracted services be competitively bid at least at intervals of three years. The impact of this action on the success of DPH applications for funds and the level of community-based organization support for such applications has not yet been assessed. It is clear, however, that the Health Commission's action has the *potential* for undermining the sense of a full partnership between the Department and cooperating community-based organizations. This potential stems largely from the environment created by formal bidding procedures, rather than from the concept of periodical review of basic partnership commitments.

SUMMARY

This chapter underscores the need for strong partnerships between the local department of public health and organizations with roots in the communities and subcultures most heavily affected by the HIV epidemic. It identifies four critical junctures at which the commitment to such partnerships has been tested during the first eight years of San Francisco's response to the epidemic.

Lessons from San Francisco: Principles of Program Design

Ron Stall, Chuck Frutchey,
Mindy Thompson Fullilove
and Pat Christen

INTRODUCTION

Designers of early San Francisco programs were eclectic in borrowing ideas from a number of communications and behavior change theories. Comprised of community organizers, public health officials, behavioral scientists and communications and marketing specialists, program designers also did considerable theorizing on their own. More than anything, these men and women were pragmatic: Time could not be spent waiting for careful, scientific studies to determine prevention strategies. Effective prevention programs were needed immediately if San Francisco's gay community was to survive. Much of the HIV prevention work done in other communities within San Francisco, specifically work with injection drug users, was undertaken under this same set of circumstances.

The following prevention principles grew out of these program experiences.

DESIGNING APPROACHES AND MESSAGES

*   *Information Itself Does Not Reduce Risk.*

When the first widespread HIV prevention campaign was being initiated in San Francisco in 1984, survey data revealed that gay and bisexual men had remarkably accurate information about how the HIV virus was transmitted.[1] Nonetheless, substantial proportions of gay men were still continuing to engage in unprotected anal intercourse at that time.

It was clear that knowledge of how to reduce the risk of HIV infection was not leading to behavior change for most gay men. Knowledge of the behavioral mechanisms by which HIV infection is spread is an absolutely necessary, but not sufficient, condition for behavior change.

*   *Be Clear About Which Behaviors Must Be Changed.*

Historically, there has been disagreement and inconsistency with regard to the behaviors that HIV prevention campaigns have sought to modify. For example, with regard to sexual transmission of HIV infection, some have argued that it is more effective to seek a reduction in the number or type of sexual partners, while others contend that campaigns should seek to encourage safe sex without regard to number or kind of sexual partners. Other questions have included whether unprotected anal or vaginal intercourse should be the sole focus of prevention campaigns or whether other sexual behaviors should also be targeted.

Regarding injection drug use, a prominent issue has concerned whether prevention workers should seek to induce a drug-free lifestyle among needle users or only to encourage cessation of needle sharing. On the broadest level, arguments have also been made that prevention campaigns would be most effective if they sought to eliminate homophobia and the combined effects of racism, sexism and poverty, as these are theoretical causes of continued high-risk sex between men, and injection drug users and their partners.

Lack of clarity in determining behaviors to be changed hampers the effectiveness of prevention efforts, because behaviors carry different meanings for individuals. For example, convincing someone to use a condom carries a completely different implication for changing behavior than does the suggestion that decreasing the number of sexual partners (or changing the kinds of sexual partners) will best lower HIV risk. Similarly, the message that HIV risk reduction is best achieved by not sharing contaminated needles holds different implications for an individual's behavior than does the message that abstinence from injection drug use is required.

Without clarity of and consensus on the messages that will result in the greatest reduction of HIV transmission, the effectiveness of HIV prevention campaigns will be compromised. The identification of specific behaviors that represent the greatest risk for HIV transmission within a community should be decided among those affected and those charged with developing HIV prevention strategies on the local level.

- *Change Group Norms to Change Individual Behaviors.*

In addition to improving knowledge levels, San Francisco program designers sought to change beliefs thought to be associated with risky behavior for HIV transmission. Specifically, they set out to convince gay men of their susceptibility to infection. They also encouraged trust in the efficacy of risk-reduction guidelines at a time when many did not believe that HIV was the causative agent or even that the virus was transmitted sexually. Prevention campaigns also persuaded individuals that they were capable of making changes and, more importantly, that enormous changes were already taking place within the community.

To understand the reasons program designers found it so important to focus on beliefs about health, community norms and gay identity, the social and historical context that provided the underpinnings of the response of the gay community to AIDS must be examined. Much has been said about the way in which the sexual lifestyle of the gay community in the 1970s and early 1980s furnished an all-too-fertile ground for the rapid spread of HIV. Likewise, it is just as important to recognize that HIV risk-reduction efforts also were shaped by the gay social institutions of the 1980s and 1990s.[2]

To many program designers, it became clear that if lives were to be saved, a redefinition of the gay male identity would have to be negotiated. No longer would it be possible for gay men to perceive their identity in sexual terms alone. A redefined identity for gay men would have to be restricted to safe sex practices and include a sense of responsibility for one's self as well as the gay community. Campaign planners recognized that changes of this nature had to be generated from within the gay male community. If they were imposed from without, there would be resistance, conflict and most damaging, delays in bringing about the changes in behavior. New norms were needed to replace old norms, but they had to be gay-positive and community-affirming. San Francisco program designers recognized the social basis of HIV risk behaviors and viewed HIV prevention as a social change process.

Recognizing the social basis of risk behaviors is important, regardless of the population being targeted for intervention. Prevention campaigns aimed at injection drug users must, for example, attempt to alter an environment that sanctions the sharing of dirty needles. As with gay men, change will be most effectively generated from within the needle-using population and must meet the unique needs of members of this community.

•   *Use Multiple Delivery Mechanisms and Peer Networks to Facilitate Risk Reduction.*

The San Francisco experience indicates that it is a mistake to rely on any one communication mechanism to effect changes in behavior. The use of a series of distinct community-wide prevention approaches working together in a synergistic fashion has the highest likelihood of reducing risk-taking behaviors within a community as a whole. Further, it has been learned that prevention messages are most effective when they are aimed at changing behaviors and beliefs at the level of peer networks.

In San Francisco, four different communication mechanisms were used to effect behavioral change within peer networks.* Media campaigns were used in the first attempt and have been used consistently throughout the epidemic. Almost all possible media outlets have been used in San Francisco, including print advertising, radio and television public service announcements, billboard and transit displays, direct mail, brochures and other printed material.

---

* The list of mechanisms is somewhat different from those in Chapter 4, reflecting the diversity of the authors' conceptualizations.

A second mechanism involved professional counseling and health education programs that directly delivered HIV prevention messages to individuals at high risk. Having such individuals participate in peer-to-peer interventions was intended to reach those who were not participants in a particular program. That is, nonparticipating peers could be reached through the unstructured process of communication and role modeling that naturally takes place within informal groups. These kinds of interventions have been particularly useful among drug users, although they also are useful for individuals referred from HIV alternative test sites, STD treatment facilities and family planning clinics.

For drug users not in treatment, the CHOW (Community Health Outreach Workers) program was developed. CHOWs were trained in "AIDS 101" and in safe needle use and sexual practices. These workers, who were former addicts, then went to areas where needle users congregate to educate them on their home turf, as well as to distribute appropriate health education materials, bleach for sterilization of needles, and condoms.

The AIDS hotline, a centralized telephone information and referral system, was the third communication mechanism. Hotlines provide easy and anonymous access to prevention information tailored to the unique needs of each individual. The stigmas associated with AIDS and the need of high-risk and/or highly fearful people to get more detailed answers to their questions than can be provided by print and electronic media make hotlines invaluable to HIV prevention efforts.

San Francisco program designers went a step further than had been attempted in most disease prevention efforts by adding a fourth communication mechanism: formal, structured interventions that emphasized interpersonal peer-to-peer communication. This approach, specifically designed to work in a structured group setting, was exemplified by the STOP AIDS Project. The STOP AIDS Project was based on survey data indicating that gay and bisexual men had been immobilized by the conflict between the growing threat of AIDS to their well-being and the sexual values and expectations characteristic of the gay subculture. This intervention was designed to promote peer support for safe sex activities and to foster peer pressure against high-risk behaviors, thereby altering community or group norms. The STOP AIDS intervention involves inviting people to participate in small group meetings held in the homes of community members to discuss personal commitment and individual actions related to ending the HIV epidemic.

• *Use Culturally Appropriate Language and Messages.*

HIV prevention messages are interpreted through the cultural lenses of those receiving them. Language comprehension is probably the most obvious and immediate factor influencing how a message is received. There are many individuals who do not know the meaning of terms such as intercourse, vagina, semen, hypodermic, condom or penis. Likewise, there are many people who do not understand terms like rimming, fisting or water sports. Clarity and understandability are basic to the development of effective HIV prevention messages.

Cultural appropriateness is also important. Overly technical language, unusual or stilted grammar and style and even slang in the wrong context can convey unintended meanings and limit the persuasiveness of messages.

Messages should relate to the experiences of target audiences. If a message talks about situations individuals have no familiarity with, it may be rejected as irrelevant or inconsequential. If a message relates to risks that clearly are relevant to some other population but not to the recipient's, that message will likely be ignored.

BUILDING RELATIONSHIPS WITH TARGET AUDIENCES

• *Define Target Audiences.*

Discussions of targeting messages are full of references to "risk groups" and "communities" when, in fact, peer groups may be the social group most relevant for purposes of educating about behavior change. Nothing has confused HIV prevention program planners more fundamentally than the lack of clarity about how to define target audiences or groups that are in need of interventions to change risky behaviors. Media commentators and policymakers, for example, have paid great attention to the concept of risk groups ever since the

Centers for Disease Control (CDC) first identified HIV infection among the populations of homosexual men, intravenous drug users and Haitians. As a result, more of an emphasis was placed on "who you are" rather than "what behaviors you engage in."

The unsophisticated use of risk group terminology can also lead to the misapplication of HIV prevention resources. For example, a sexually active Black teenage girl may have more in common with a sexually active Hispanic teenage girl than with some other members of her own race. Therefore, programs that are targeted to teens may be more effective in changing the behavior of Black teens than programs aimed at Black populations as a whole.

The language of HIV prevention is also replete with references to "communities," when in fact, many of the target audiences for programs are not communities. It is unlikely, for example, that sexual partners of injection drug users are a community. They may share important demographic characteristics and behaviors that put them at risk, but they are not communities in the sense of sharing a common identification and affiliation. For this reason, it may be useful to establish formal organizations when none exist within targeted populations. On the other hand, when there are existing community-based organizations, it may make sense to work with these groups and through their networks to reach audiences.

The literature on the formation of group norms assigns particular importance to peer groups. It is through such peer groups that norms are changed. Hence, if norms are an important focus of HIV prevention efforts, target audiences should be defined with respect to these peer groups. Moreover, the definition of target audiences should be based on knowledge, attitude and behavior surveys conducted in each locale where programs are being started. These surveys have been critical to the design of programs in San Francisco and are discussed more fully later.

- *Understand the Beliefs of Target Audiences.*

The meaning of the HIV epidemic and of risk behaviors varies greatly among different target audiences for HIV prevention programs. For example, the perceived risk from AIDS may arouse less fear among injection drug users whose lifestyle includes, by definition, numerous life-threatening risks. On the other hand, the anguish

104

associated with premature death may arouse deep fear among middle-class gay men who have not been accustomed to facing their own mortality. In one target audience, to cite another example, a woman carrying a condom is regarded as sophisticated; this same behavior could label the woman as a prostitute if she were a member of a different target audience.

Descriptive research of target audiences is needed before messages and communication strategies are finalized. This research should focus on the size and demographic composition of the audience as well as on the geographic distribution of audience members. Most importantly, it should examine the meaning of the epidemic and of risk behaviors within the cultural context of each group.

• *Involve Representatives from Target Audiences.*

Individuals either from the target audiences or who understand and are respectful of the values and cultures of those audiences should be actively involved in all levels of the design and implementation of HIV prevention campaigns.

Representatives from the target group should be carefully chosen. No one person can fully represent the interests, values and outlooks of any target group. For this reason, it is best to have a number of different representatives of the target group. It is also invaluable to have representation of people who are similar to the target group populations at all planning phases. On the other hand, it can be problematic for any group to be too homogeneous, as "outsiders" can also have vitally important insights. Public health personnel and behavioral scientists involved in program design should view themselves as catalysts and facilitators rather than as leaders of prevention campaigns. Whenever possible, professional researchers also should be drawn from the target groups or communities.

Focus groups provide an excellent setting to get feedback on a project while it is in development. Additional representatives of the target group (who are not involved with the project) can give "off-the-street" feedback on the project's appropriateness, potential interest and potential effectiveness. They can also suggest new directions for the project or provide valuable ideas for future projects.

It is important to recognize that political leaders and traditionally defined gatekeepers are not always members of the peer groups that need to be targeted for HIV prevention campaigns. If it is important to reach teenagers, for example, then *teenagers* must play a crucial role in the planning process. In this instance, adult gatekeepers have a role to play, but teenagers must be recruited and given leadership positions within teen prevention campaigns.

• *Be Sensitive to Target Audiences.*

Many of those affected most directly by the HIV epidemic have survived long histories of discrimination within American society. Some of the justification for discrimination has to do with precisely those sexual and drug-using behaviors that are implicated in HIV transmission, thus making prevention efforts especially delicate.

Attempts to involve populations with a history of discrimination must then be very sensitive to issues of social stigma. Lack of sensitivity can suggest that public health personnel want to prolong a group's struggle for acceptance. The widespread perception that an agency is insensitive to issues of stigmatization and/or discrimination will hinder prevention efforts by that agency.

Thus, through continued contact with members of affected target groups, both on a staff and personal level, a fuller understanding of the conditions under which risk for HIV continues to occur can be reached. Through insights achieved through direct contact and working relationships forged with members of target populations, the effectiveness of prevention efforts can be magnified.

• *Make AIDS Relevant to Affected Populations.*

In many communities or target populations, HIV prevention is not the only serious issue. Gay men have concerns regarding homophobia and discrimination. Ethnic populations face poverty, drug abuse and other social problems, including discrimination. In this context, HIV prevention must compete with many other issues for people's attention. Strategies that link AIDS to other community problems may increase the likelihood of HIV prevention becoming and remaining a salient issue. Nevertheless, San Francisco program designers have attempted to keep interventions focused on prevention efforts that primarily attempt to change risky behaviors and thus reduce the risk of transmission of HIV.

CHANGING PUBLIC POLICY

* *Advocate for Necessary Changes in Laws and Institutions.*

To achieve maximum effectiveness, HIV prevention efforts may require advocacy of legal and institutional change. For example, to be effective, HIV prevention messages must be clear and explicit about sexual and drug-using practices that place individuals at risk of infection. Yet, designers of prevention programs have faced prohibitions on the use of federal and state funds for dissemination of explicit messages. Also, needle exchanges are illegal in many areas of the United States, although they may be effective in limiting the spread of HIV infection among needle-injecting drug users. It is commonplace for those who wish to prevent the spread of HIV infection to be confronted with continued legal, political and as a result, funding restrictions.

Public health leaders, health professionals and AIDS service providers must be prepared to advocate legal and institutional changes supportive of educational efforts to change high-risk behavior.

RESEARCH AND EVALUATION

* *Develop Partnerships that Link Research and Action.*

The San Francisco model of HIV prevention has come to be synonymous with the idea of partnership between public health authorities and community-based groups. As has been pointed out, the Department of Public Health actively involved gay men early in the process of designing and implementing risk reduction programs. Today, the Department is involving ethnic populations and women in the same way.

The link between research and action has been equally important in San Francisco. Research helped to drive the process of intervention design and implementation. As interventions have been put in place, new questions have been generated to be explored in subsequent research. The results have led to refinements in programs. This process has been greatly strengthened through the active collaboration of public health authorities, AIDS service providers and communications, social science and behavioral researchers.

- **Become Familiar with Models and Theories of Behavior Change.**

Many prevention programs are attempted without any reference to models or theory. As a result, program planners all too often fail to grapple with critical questions: What emphasis should be given to knowledge-enhancing messages at a particular stage of the epidemic? How important is the belief in personal efficacy, the idea that one has the ability to successfully initiate and sustain changes in behavior? Do certain skills need to be acquired? If so, which ones are most important?

The adoption of any specific theory of behavior change is not being advocated here. In fact, there is no validated model of sexual or drug-using behavior change. Program designers should become familiar with leading theoretical perspectives. They should think clearly and rigorously about the behaviors to be influenced and the factors that might influence them. Without insights drawn from these theoretical perspectives, it is highly doubtful that campaigns can succeed.

Familiarity with leading theories of risk reduction allows program designers to build programs that support needed behavioral changes. Through experimentation with different approaches with distinct populations, it can more quickly be learned which approaches to supporting risk reduction are most effective. This is true, however, only if variables are carefully specified, measured and analyzed in evaluations of these approaches.

It is easy to misinterpret this appeal for theorizing and evaluation as a call for research at the expense of action. Nothing could be more antithetical to the experience of San Francisco. Program planners in the city put the emphasis on action, on the rapid deployment of intervention in an effort to save lives. Creativity and innovation were encouraged. There was also, however, a respect for what had been learned in other health behavior change efforts and a conviction that action should be based on the best, most careful and rigorous thinking possible.

- **Understand Why Individuals Continue to Take Risks.**

Within all target audiences, some individuals successfully adopt new, lower risk behaviors and maintain them consistently over time. Others never initiate new behaviors but continue high-risk practices. A third group moves back and forth—sometimes practicing lower-risk behaviors and sometimes reverting to high-risk behaviors. This third group is critically important to the effort to control the epidemic. It is urgent that program designers understand the distinctions between those people who continue to maintain adopted behavior changes over the long haul and those who do not.[3]

In San Francisco, ongoing surveys have made possible the identification of individuals who lapse in their commitment to practice only safe behaviors. Within the gay male audience, for example, surveys have found that relapse from safe sex seems to be highly structured by relationship status. Among gay men in stable relationships, having the same antibody status and "being in love" were the reasons given for having unprotected anal intercourse. Men not involved in such relationships report reasons for having unprotected anal intercourse that are more circumstantial in nature and are not derived from the needs associated with a well-defined relationship (i.e., being "turned on," the combination of sex with alcohol or drugs, not having any condoms available at the time).

• *Use Multiple Tools for Evaluation.*

San Francisco program designers have found it critical to evaluate programs and to assess the degree of behavior change. Several different evaluation techniques have been used to determine the effectiveness of prevention techniques in the effort to continue to shape the scope and directions of HIV prevention programs.[4]

Standard process evaluation techniques have been used to determine how many high-risk individuals are being reached, whether interventions are efficiently delivered and the level of client satisfaction with programs and services.

Advertising research techniques have been used to determine the reach and penetration of campaign messages. Message awareness and recall data have been regularly collected. Planners also have examined the relationship between message acceptance and attitude and behavior change. On this score, there is evidence that acceptance of prevention campaign messages has been associated with behavior change.

Regular knowledge, attitude and behavior studies have been conducted among gay and bisexual men, multiple/high-risk partner heterosexuals, drug users and members of ethnic groups at heightened risk of HIV infection. Most of the studies have been conducted on a population basis using either telephone or in-person interviewing techniques.

SUMMARY

The strategy for risk reduction in San Francisco was eclectic in nature, emphasizing pragmatic approaches to risk reduction over theoretical considerations. Emphasis was placed on developing a public health strategy, with considerable latitude given to experiment with interventions that could result in "failures." Further, considerable weight was given to qualitative, focus group data (in which members of target populations were directly interviewed with open-ended questions) as a means of devising and testing specific prevention approaches.

For these reasons, many divergent approaches to behavioral risk reduction are represented in the prevention model. Theoretical approaches included an amalgamation of standard behavioral interventions (raising levels of AIDS health knowledge and concern, attempts to raise levels of personal efficacy and attempts to diffuse risk reduction techniques within the community) and interventions that were more unusual in the public health field (community organizing, social marketing and attempts to induce changes in group norms concerning risk-taking behaviors).

As HIV prevention efforts seek to reach populations in other communities, the San Francisco experience indicates that direct community participation, continued use of divergent theoretical approaches, reliance on behavioral research and the use of innovative communication mechanisms will be necessary if the spread of HIV infection is to be stopped.

Part III
HIV Prevention in Your Community

7

Planning and Implementing Community Strategies

Pat Franks, Henrik L. Blum,
Thomas J. Coates, Edward S. Morales
and Paul M. Gibson

INTRODUCTION

Planning is a way for people to think things through, to work things through and to get things done. Planning and implementing integrated, community-wide HIV prevention strategies have posed problems for cities and counties in the United States for several reasons. First, there has been no national consensus about what HIV prevention approaches and messages should be used to reach different audiences. For the most part, effective working relationships have not been formed among federal, state and local levels of government and with community-based groups and other private sector groups in terms of HIV prevention priorities, policies, programs and funding. Second, there has been no widescale national demonstration program to support the development of comprehensive, community-wide HIV prevention strategies. Third, communities themselves have experienced serious difficulties in building consensus for HIV prevention efforts. Fourth, most community experiments in HIV prevention have not been evaluated, and there is little information to guide communities about what works and what does not work with different populations in halting the spread of HIV infection.

This chapter examines the general response of communities to the HIV epidemic, factors influencing community response, stages in community response, the role of community planning in relation to HIV prevention, different types of planning for different purposes and 12 basic steps in the planning and implementation process at the community level. The chapter concludes with some words about the importance of different types of evaluation.

LEVELS OF COMMUNITY RESPONSE

Response to the HIV epidemic has evolved through a "bottoms up" rather than a "top down" process of planning, program development and policy development. Cities and counties were the first to be challenged to respond to the epidemic, and they were the first to experiment with different approaches to HIV prevention, care and support. During 1981 and 1982, nearly 80 percent of all reported AIDS cases were in six metropolitan areas—New York City, San Francisco, Los Angeles, Miami, Newark and Houston.[1] Faced with rapidly increasing numbers of AIDS cases and fears about the spread of this new disease, concerned people in some of these areas began, in 1983 and 1984, to launch experiments to prevent further HIV infection among populations most at risk and to define and develop elements of a continuum of care and support for people with AIDS. In other areas, local leadership was slow to emerge, and response to the epidemic lagged behind.

Local response to the epidemic has resulted in the development of distinct HIV prevention approaches for different populations. Examples of approaches that began in high-impact communities and are now being used in many communities include: STOP AIDS-type projects for homosexual/bisexual men; "soap opera" educational videos for Hispanic adults; comic books, fotonovelas and rap contests for Black and Hispanic teens; innovative peer-based school curricula for teens; bleach education projects using former addicts as community health outreach workers to teach injection drug users to flush their works; and the use of female peer counselors to reach partners of injection drug users.

Comprehensive, integrated, community-wide HIV prevention strategies, however, have been slow in evolving. The Centers for Disease Control (CDC), other federal agencies, and state and local government agencies have funded projects directed toward the development of school-based projects, projects directed toward ethnic minorities, drug abuse-related projects and other community-based projects. However, federal and state constraints on the content of prevention and education materials and on nontraditional prevention approaches have hindered communities in developing prevention programs. Private sector support of HIV prevention efforts has involved both private foundation and corporate efforts. However, in most cases, these efforts have not encouraged risk taking in developing programs.

Communities also have faced problems in developing consensus and support for HIV prevention efforts. As a result, programs have been slow to evolve. The development time from planning and start-up to funding and implementation is long, often several years. Evaluation also continues to be a problem. There is as yet little evidence regarding the effectiveness of specific interventions in specific populations. Evaluation of multiple-intervention, community-wide HIV prevention approaches, even more difficult and costly, has not begun.

By 1990 more than two dozen major metropolitan areas in the United States had been seriously affected by the HIV epidemic.[2] The impact of the epidemic has intensified sharply in cities that were the original epicenters, and it has expanded to other major metropolitan areas, as well as to smaller cities, suburban areas and rural areas. Only 40 percent of cumulative reported AIDS cases are now reported from San Francisco and other cities first impacted by the epidemic.[3]

More and more communities are now under pressure to plan, organize, deliver and develop financing strategies for a broader array of HIV prevention, care and support services. As the number of persons with HIV disease continues to increase, as more people fall ill and as the clinical management of HIV infection shifts further toward early intervention, localities are being faced with a complex task. This task is to integrate public health services (e.g., HIV testing and counseling) with education programs (e.g., peer-based and other HIV prevention efforts), personal health services (e.g., diagnostic testing and monitoring, primary care services and drug treatment), social services, home- and community-based services, outpatient substance abuse treatment services, residential care (e.g., substance abuse and mental health) and housing. Cities and counties will likely continue to be the planners and program developers of first and last resort in the HIV epidemic.

FACTORS THAT INFLUENCE COMMUNITY RESPONSE

A number of factors influence community response to the HIV epidemic. It is important to understand how these factors interact in shaping a community's response, particularly in terms of the community's readiness and capacity to develop HIV prevention strategies.

The general factors influencing community response are:

• the perceived magnitude and seriousness of the HIV epidemic in the community, including the cumulative number of reported AIDS cases, the number of AIDS deaths and seroprevalence rates in different populations;

• the populations most affected by HIV disease and the populations at risk of HIV infection;

• the modes of transmission of HIV infection;

• the availability, or lack of availability, of effective HIV prevention interventions and effective treatments for HIV disease;

• the cost of HIV prevention interventions, as well as the costs of treatment, care and support for persons with HIV disease;

• the role of government agencies, including intergovernmental relations (i.e., the relationship of federal, state, county and municipal levels of government) and the relationship of the public sector to the

private sector, particularly the nonprofit voluntary sector, in terms of priority setting, policy development and resource allocation for HIV prevention, treatment, care and support services;
 • the economic health of the community;
 • the social health of the community, particularly its response to other emergencies, crises and social and health problems; and
 • public attitudes, beliefs and biases about HIV disease and the groups most affected by the disease.

A major factor influencing community response to the HIV epidemic is the role played by county and municipal government, particularly the leadership role of elected officials and public health officials. Other significant factors include the leadership roles of health care professionals and health education specialists and individuals and groups most directly affected by the epidemic, including persons with AIDS and persons at risk of HIV infection, gay and lesbian advocacy and service organizations and ethnic minority advocacy and service organizations. Still other factors include the specific roles played by others in the private sector, including businesses, churches and synagogues, community service organizations, private foundations and the media. The abundance or lack of community resources and services, including health and human service agencies and schools, colleges and universities, will also affect community response. Finally, the presence or absence of functional forums for community-wide priority setting, problem solving and planning related to health and social problems, including both the public and private sectors, will affect response.

STAGES IN COMMUNITY RESPONSE

Community response to the HIV epidemic often proceeds in stages. These stages can be compared to some of the stages observed in individuals' responses to their own HIV infection. For example, Elisabeth Kubler-Ross and others have described several distinct stages in the response of persons to their knowledge that they have been infected and to their experience of living—and dying—with HIV disease. These stages include denial and isolation, anger, bargaining, depression and acceptance.[4]

In observing communities, four stages of response can be identified. Stage 1, the initial response, is denial. Stage 2 is characterized by struggle and sometimes panic. Stage 3 signals a move toward acceptance and coping. Stage 4 signals "relapse" and return to struggle. Not all communities go through all stages. Nor do communities necessarily go through the stages in a strict linear fashion, proceeding from one stage to the next over specific and predictable time periods.

Stage 1: Denial

This stage is characterized by widespread lack of community awareness or community agreement that the HIV epidemic is a community problem. During this stage, there are initial attempts, usually of a relatively few individuals—public health leaders, health professionals, members of the gay and lesbian community, members of ethnic communities, business or religious leaders, political leaders or those in the media—*to raise the visibility of HIV disease in the community*. Service components may begin to be developed and services provided, but they are insufficient to meet growing needs. Care, treatment and support services are usually developed before HIV prevention programs, because the demand for these services is more apparent and more readily justified. Also, there are usually fewer value conflicts among community members about how to proceed with developing and providing these services. Service and advocacy groups, often with a volunteer base and supported by private donations, may emerge to try to fill service gaps in some communities. In other communities, no such efforts may arise. This stage, which is usually difficult, may also be prolonged, lasting several years.

Stage 2: Struggle

This stage is characterized by continuing attempts to raise the visibility of HIV disease as a community issue and *to validate or to legitimize HIV disease as a community problem* requiring the allocation of local public resources or a search for public or private resources outside the community. The decision to allocate local resources is usually a turning point in the community's response to the epidemic. The decision to seek public or private resources outside the community from the CDC, the Health Resources and Services Administration, state agencies or a private foundation also represents an important trigger point in community response. This is especially true if a Request For Proposal (RFP) has been issued, asking the community to respond by developing a plan of action for a pilot project or community-wide demonstration project. This "carrot" may enhance cooperation among groups in the community. It also may create hostility as public and private agencies vie among themselves for control of the planning process and for control of specific arenas of activity and dollars.

This phase is usually marked by confrontations, often hostile and polarizing, among public sector agencies and between public and private sector groups, particularly advocacy groups, about issues of responsibility for growing problems and needs related to the epidemic. At this time, there are initial attempts to assess needs and to inventory resources. Again, this stage may last a considerable time, sometimes several years. During this stage, the epidemic frequently gets ahead of the community response in terms of numbers and needs. Again, HIV prevention and education efforts may lose out to care, treatment and support services in terms of the allocation of resources.

Stage 3: Acceptance and Coping

This stage is characterized by community "ownership" of HIV disease as a legitimate community problem. There are more systematic attempts *to assess needs and to plan, organize, develop and provide a more complete continuum of HIV prevention, care and support services*. There are also conscious attempts to develop a service delivery system, as well to develop at least a short-term financing strategy to support different service components. There also may be calls for research and for evaluation of pilot programs or demonstration programs launched earlier. Strong public health and medical and nursing leadership appear to be essential ingredients in this process, as does the involvement of persons with AIDS and persons at risk of HIV infection. The degree of cooperation between public and private sector groups during all stages of a community's response, but especially during this stage, is another critical factor in the models of HIV prevention, care and support developed, the comprehensiveness of the system and the approach to financing services. There are different levels of coping, some more successful than others and some more future oriented than others.

Stage 4: Relapse

Communities can slip back from a coping stage into a struggle stage because of increasing AIDS cases in the face of decreasing resources, and because of competing community health and social problems and increased competition for resources. All of the characteristics of the struggle stage may be reactivated during the relapse stage, including hostile and polarizing confrontations about relative needs, responsibilities and resource allocations. Blame laying and finger pointing, especially at other levels of government, are common. Groups advocating for other causes and concerns are often pitted against AIDS advocacy groups and against local government officials supporting AIDS programs and funding. Groups supporting HIV prevention and education efforts also may be pitted against groups supporting HIV care, treatment and support services. There may well be more insistent calls for research and evaluation related to HIV prevention to determine whether what has been done is really working.

Looking back over the first decade of the HIV epidemic, it appears that an unplanned, haphazard political response is generated when AIDS concerns are raised in a given community. First, activists try to alert the community about the health threat. Second, factions within the public or private sectors respond by applying political pressure and by mobilizing resources without widespread community input or a formal planning process. Third, experiments, including pilot and demonstration projects, are proposed, attempted and sometimes funded by government or private sources. Fourth, there is a call for evaluation and research. Fifth, programs are refined and further developed with or without the benefit of information gained from evaluation. Sixth, policies are developed and comprehensive community planning is finally initiated. This process has repeated itself in many communities in relation to the HIV epidemic. Communities affected later in the epidemic appear to be reliving the experience of communities first affected by the epidemic.

DEVELOPING STRATEGIES: THE ROLE OF PLANNING

Community planning is an activity that involves exploring the major value systems of a community, finding out how these values shape a community's concerns, discovering what the community regards as problems and then clarifying what the community has available and will accept in terms of solutions for the problems it identifies. For example, a community may identify the spread of HIV infection as a problem. A majority of people in the community also may understand that there are clear-cut epidemiologic pathways, such as the role of sexual behavior and injection drug use in the transmission of HIV infection, that point the way to interventions that might help solve the problem. However, effective interventions to change sexual behavior or drug-using behavior may not be available because they have not yet been developed and tested or because they may not be acceptable to many groups in the community.

In a democracy, diversity in values, and occasionally even serious conflict in values, is to be expected. The political adjustment of major value disagreements among groups is a critical feature of a reasonably functioning community, state or nation in a democratic society. Therefore, seeking to encourage the respectful engagement of people with different values in identifying problems and in proposing potential solutions to problems is a major consideration of community planning.

Community planning must take into account four basic tenets:

• Each community has distinctive features that characterize the nature of a problem, for example, the spread of HIV infection.

• No two communities have the same array of involved individuals or groups.

• Demographic and epidemiologic data are necessary to clarify the nature of the problem, but other information, including ethnographic information, information about other attempts to change individual behavior and community norms and information about community dynamics, also is necessary.

• A high level of political awareness is the key to planning that has as its goal community-legitimated action that effectively solves the problem tackled.

Different types of planning can be used by communities for different purposes, as communities proceed from developing broad policy goals to implementing specific programs related to HIV prevention and education.[5]

Policy Planning

The purpose of policy planning is to answer the question: *What should we do?* At this level, planning is goal oriented. People are trying to figure out in a broad sense how to respond to a problem. Often, they are trying to create new interventions in response to a new problem, such as the spread of HIV infection. Here technical information, such as demographic, epidemiologic, health systems, health manpower and cost data, is helpful in describing the nature and extent of the problem, as well as some of the potential solutions. Information about the groups most affected by the problem and their views about how to deal with the problem is essential. For example, convening focus groups of gay men or injection drug users to discuss the spread of HIV infection and ways to stop it is a necessary first step in developing HIV prevention strategies directed toward these groups. It is also important to have information about how institutions in the community are organized to respond, how the system works and does not work and who does what. It helps too, to know what other people are doing to solve the problem—for example, what HIV prevention interventions are being tried in different populations by people in other communities. The outcome of this type of planning is often a statement of goals or priorities and recommendations about how they should be met.

Strategic Planning

The purpose of strategic planning is to answer the question: *What can we do?* At this level, planning is objective oriented. People are trying to develop specific objectives related to their goals and to explore different strategies for achieving them. For example, a major objective of HIV prevention and education efforts may be to reduce rates of new infection in specific target populations. Here, information about opportunities and constraints, costs and benefits and efficiency and effectiveness, including cost effectiveness, of different interventions is critical. Information from evaluations of different HIV prevention interventions in different populations in achieving specific objectives is invaluable.

Tactical, Operational or Implementation Planning

The purpose of this type of planning is to answer the question: *What will we do?* At this level, planning is action oriented. People decide not only what they will do, but also how they will do it, who will do it, when it will be done, how much it will cost and how to measure, monitor and evaluate the results. Here, tasks, methods and procedures, responsibilities, timelines, costs, anticipated effects or outcomes and monitoring and evaluation are laid out.

One of the major challenges of planning at all levels is to build as broad a consensus as possible in the community. Without some degree of consensus about the nature and extent of the problem and what to do about it, no plan will work. To build consensus, representatives of all groups that are affected by the problem—that have a stake in the problem—and that will have responsibility for solving it must be invited and involved, at some point, to participate in the planning process.

Since individual behavior change and changes in community norms of behavior are critical to HIV prevention efforts, persons who are HIV-infected, persons at risk of infection and groups serving persons with HIV infection must be involved from the start in all levels of the community planning process. As it becomes clear that other groups will have a role to play in determining the extent of the problem and potential solutions, they, too, must be included in the planning process.

COMMUNITY PLANNING: TWELVE BASIC STEPS

1. *Convene a preplanning HIV focus group.* This group should include six to ten people who are known to be well informed about HIV disease. The expertise of the group should encompass: (a) epidemiologic knowledge and skills; (b) political skills; (c) clinical skills related to preventing, diagnosing and treating HIV infection; (d) behavioral and social science skills; (e) community organizing skills; (f) persons with HIV infection or persons at risk of HIV infection; (g) representatives of local AIDS service or education organizations; and (h) a person with formal planning skills in community process settings. The group should include people of different racial/ethnic, socioeconomic and religious backgrounds, as well as people of different sexual orientations and gender.*

2. *Engage the preplanning HIV focus group in an analysis of the problem—the spread of HIV infection in the community.* The first task of the group is to describe the nature and scope of the problem in the community, including precursors to the problem and consequences of the problem.

3. *Ask the preplanning HIV focus group to "invent" potentially useful interventions to prevent the spread of HIV infection in the community.* The second task of the group is to brainstorm what might be done about the problem by coming up with as many ways as possible to block the spread of HIV.

4. *Give the preplanning HIV focus group the assignment of ranking potentially useful interventions according to their effectiveness and technical and political feasibility.* The third task of the group is to prioritize interventions in terms of their potential effectiveness in preventing the spread of HIV infection in the community and their technical feasibility. The group should then consider how to garner community consensus in support of its top proposals.

5. *Establish an HIV Prevention Planning Task Force to develop a priority list of interventions for the community.* Broad-based, community-wide task forces have been used effectively by many communities to set priorities, to develop plans of action and to achieve

---

* For a more complete discussion of community health planning see H.L. Blum, *Planning for Health*, Human Sciences Press, N.Y., 1989, especially 225-262.

consensus in the community about developing HIV prevention, care and support services. Task forces are often established by mayors' offices or by county commissioners or boards of supervisors. The task force should be inclusive, rather than exclusive, in its membership. It can include as few as 25 members or as many as 150 members organized into special task force work groups.

The HIV Prevention Planning Task Force membership should include: (a) astute "bridgers," including community organizers, respected community leaders and political, business and religious leaders; (b) experts in epidemiology, clinical medicine, nursing, behavioral medicine, substance abuse, social work, public health administration, health economics and health policy, and planning; (c) special stakeholders, including persons with HIV disease and persons with HIV infection, members of ethnic groups, members of gay and lesbian advocacy and service organizations and members of AIDS service and education organizations; (d) government agencies (federal, state and local) involved in policy setting, program administration, financing and regulation (the mayor's office, the departments of health, human services, education, police, criminal justice); and (e) private sector agencies with special interests, including insurers, health maintenance organizations, hospitals and private foundations.

The work tasks of the HIV Prevention Planning Task Force should parallel the work tasks of the preplanning HIV focus group. However, the task force will explore the problem and potential interventions in more depth.

Each of the interventions that the HIV Prevention Planning Task Force membership feels is worth exploring should be assigned to a task force work group that is authorized to obtain whatever community and expert guidance it feels is needed to determine the feasibility of a given intervention.

The following criteria can be used to prioritize interventions: (a) benefits (e.g., numbers avoiding infection, probable savings in lives, productivity, costs of care); (b) costs directly incurred in carrying out the HIV prevention intervention; (c) who gains and who loses in terms of dollars or illness; (d) availability of technology to carry out the intervention; (e) social concerns of community met or violated;

and (f) political feasibility.

6. *Encourage broad-based collaboration in the design of HIV prevention interventions.* Different groups in the community have different skills and experience to bring to the table when pilot projects reach the design stage or the nuts and bolts stage. University and community-based scientists knowledgeable about HIV infection, including epidemiologists and behavioral and social scientists, can be invaluable in helping to construct projects with specific objectives that can be measured, monitored and evaluated. Health educators working in departments of health and community-based organizations have practical experience in designing and implementing programs from the point of view of the specific tasks involved in reaching target populations and encouraging their participation. Community leaders will know whether programs will be accepted or rejected by specific populations. State and federal health officials, as well as private and corporate foundation program officers, will know if the proposed project fits current program and funding guidelines.

7. *Seek funding to implement interventions, beginning with pilot projects and demonstrations.* When dealing with a new or complex problem, there is simply no way to be sure that a proposed intervention will work. The only thing to do is to try it—to conduct a small-scale pilot project or a demonstration project. The search to obtain start-up funds for such projects should begin close to home. Local departments of health and private and corporate foundations with a community, regional or statewide focus are logical sources of funding for such projects. Turnaround time from proposal to funding is usually short, and proposal guidelines are often simple and easy to follow.

State departments of health, the CDC and the Office of Substance Abuse Prevention of the federal Alcohol, Drug Abuse and Mental Health Administration are other possible sources of funding, as are private and corporate foundations with a national focus. Foundation Centers, Funders Concerned about AIDS, the National AIDS Clearinghouse, the American Foundation for AIDS Research, local offices of state legislators and members of the U.S. Congress often can provide information about private and public sources of funding for HIV-related projects.

Do not be discouraged by initial failure to obtain funding for projects. Do what you can to set preliminary stages of the project in motion with volunteer effort and contributed resources. Learn what you can to strengthen the specific aims of the project and methods for achieving those aims. Document what you have learned, sharpen the project's focus, and try again.

8. *Monitor and evaluate the results of the intervention.* No project, however small, should be planned, designed and implemented without a plan to monitor and evaluate the project's results. Always enlist the help of persons trained in different evaluation methods to help plan, design and implement HIV prevention projects.

9. *Give feedback to the community.* Pilot projects and demonstration projects are most often launched with the enthusiastic support of a number of groups and institutions in the community. Just as often, news of the results of these projects fails to reach the very people who would most benefit from the information. People responsible for launching a project also have a responsibility to provide feedback regarding the project, not only at its end but also over its course. News releases, newsletters and special bulletins about the project's progress are good ways to keep people informed. Publication of research and evaluation findings in widely circulated, peer-reviewed journals is essential if projects are to be replicated by other communities and states. The publications are also are helpful in informing policymakers at the federal, state and local levels of government.

10. *Get feedback from the community.* A pilot or demonstration project may have been successful in achieving some of its objectives and a dismal failure in achieving other objectives. Feedback from people involved in the project, including project participants, trained evaluators and funding agencies, is invaluable in retooling project objectives or specific aspects of interventions.

11. *Refine interventions and seek funding to expand pilot programs and demonstrations to full-scale projects.* The next step in creating a community-wide HIV prevention effort is to learn from what has worked—or not worked—in pilot and demonstration projects and to move toward the development of more comprehensive programs. Some caveats are in order. First, what worked in one population may not work in another population. Second, what worked at one point in

the epidemic may not be appropriate at another point. The needs of target populations and the dimensions of the epidemic change over time. The growing importance of early intervention in HIV disease is a good example of a major change in the epidemic that requires new links among prevention, care, and support services. Third, be thoughtful and persistent and plan for long-term HIV efforts that are integrated with other disease prevention, health prevention and primary health care programs in the community. The HIV epidemic is not going to end tomorrow. In fact, if the spread of HIV infection is to be substantially curtailed, HIV prevention efforts will need to continue with stable sources of public and private sector funding.

12. *Continue to experiment.* New groups, particularly children and youth, will need to be reached with new HIV approaches and messages as the epidemic continues. There is a great and continuing need for innovative approaches that address sexual and drug-taking behaviors that put young people at risk of HIV infection. There is also a need for innovative approaches in populations such as gay and bisexual men, who have already been reached with initial HIV prevention and education messages but who are experiencing difficulties in sustaining behavior change over the long term. Without continued experimentation—and evaluation—at the community level, the challenge of preventing the spread of HIV infection will not be met.

THE IMPORTANCE OF EVALUATION

Evaluation is a systemic process that produces a trustworthy account of what was attempted and why. Through the examination of results—the outcomes of intervention programs—it answers the questions: What was done? To whom and how? and What outcomes were observed? Well-designed evaluations permit drawing inferences from data and address the difficult question: What do the outcomes mean? Well-executed evaluations provide credible information about program effectiveness.[6]

There are many aspects or versions of evaluation. Some of the more useful types of evaluation are reviewed below.

Formative evaluation: This is the first effort at evaluation. It occurs after program design but before implementation of a program. Formative evaluations are relatively small-scale efforts to identify evaluation issues before a program is implemented. Examples of strategies to be used here are interviews, focus groups, surveys and pilot studies of interventions. For example, in formulating a program to reduce HIV-related high-risk behavior among adolescents, the program developers might want to conduct surveys to determine what kinds of behaviors adolescents engage in frequently, which they prefer and the determinants of both. Program developers also might want to conduct focus groups and interviews with selected adolescents to determine their individual preferences and also their ideas about program formats. A program might be developed and pilot tests conducted before final implementation. The pilot test would not require that a rigorous evaluation be conducted. Rather, additional interviews or surveys of the adolescents might be conducted to collect ideas about how to modify the program to make it more suitable for the audience.

Process evaluation: This step occurs as the program is being implemented. It seeks to answer the questions: What was done? To whom? How? Process evaluation is carried out to insure that goals and objectives are being met. The process evaluation of an advertising campaign, for example, may help to determine how many messages were delivered via which media and how many people may have been aware of or may have actually read these messages. Process evaluation may contribute information necessary to redevelop delivery strategies to retrack program objectives as the epidemic changes. Process evaluation is important but not sufficient because, while it can help to determine what was done, it cannot determine the impact achieved by any specific program or campaign.

Outcome evaluation: This form of evaluation is designed to identify the effectiveness and consequences of the program. Outcome evaluation tries to answer the questions: What outcomes were observed? What do the outcomes mean? Do the outcomes make a difference? Questions also can be asked about the potential harmful effects of programs. It is important in outcome evaluation to pay close attention to scientific principles about the measurement of outcomes, as well as to strategies for improving the designs of such evaluations. Of course, evaluators have to be alert to the presence of other forces acting at the same time that might account for the evident success or failure of the intervention (e.g., new cases might be occurring as frequently as ever not as a result of the intervention's failure, but because of heavy immigration of people with HIV disease into an area).

SUMMARY

Communities have experienced serious problems in planning and implementing integrated, community-wide HIV prevention strategies. Many of these problems stem from the lack of consensus about what HIV prevention approaches and messages should be used to reach different audiences and the lack of effective working relationships among different levels of government (federal, state, county and municipal) and private sector groups. Other problems stem from the lack of evaluation of community experiments in HIV prevention and the lack of information about what works and what does not work with different populations in halting the spread of HIV infection. Programs have been developed and launched over the course of the epidemic in an unplanned and haphazard way in an environment characterized by sharp and highly politicized conflicts.

Comprehensive community planning involves a broad array of individuals, groups and institutions with diverse skills and responsibilities working together to prioritize, design, implement and evaluate HIV prevention interventions. Collaborative planning efforts centered on problem identification, problem analysis and problem solving help to uncover value conflicts among groups and institutions and to build community-wide consensus about potentially useful interventions that may first be developed as pilot or demonstration projects and then as wider-scale programs.

Evaluation of community experiments in HIV prevention and education is a key to the development and diffusion of specific interventions for specific target populations. An adequately funded, widescale national demonstration program designed to support the development and evaluation of comprehensive, integrated, community-wide HIV prevention strategies is critically needed. Community HIV prevention strategies will need to be supported over the long term by a stable base of public and private funding, such as that provided for hypertension control and other successful disease prevention efforts. Community HIV prevention efforts will also need to be integrated into other disease prevention, health promotion and primary care programs at the local level.

8

Ending the HIV Epidemic:
A Call for Community Action

Timothy R. Wolfred

To stop AIDS is to build community.

It has been said that disease is a breakdown of community and that the cure lies in the strengthening of community. San Francisco's strategy in the HIV epidemic has been just that: to build communities when they did not exist, to bolster communities when they needed to be strengthened.

At a recent organizing conference, a leading Black health educator framed the challenge: "We want to provide education and information that will empower Black women to take control of their bodies and to become involved in a movement that helps to prevent the spread of AIDS.... It is critical that [San Francisco] Bay Area Black females, young ones in particular, become politically mobilized around AIDS."

As the second decade of the HIV epidemic arrives, HIV prevention remains a community-based movement. Efforts in San Francisco and elsewhere will continue to require bold challenges to prevailing social and group norms that would prevent our talking about such matters as anal sex and oral sex, cleaning and exchanging needles, as well as about condoms for the incarcerated or for teens. Public conflict about strategies and policies is still welcomed in San Francisco as a way to engage the entire population in a debate about HIV prevention efforts. Our partnerships with business and church leaders, with the media and with politicians and public health officials are as crucial as ever to funding our work and developing our strategies.

Our work in the 1990s continues to be fueled by the enduring passion and determination that comes from the realization that lives are at stake. Some policymakers and public health leaders have proclaimed that the epidemic has peaked; they are wrong. New infections and more and more deaths will be seen in every corner of this nation for the foreseeable future. We cannot rest yet. This "call to action" lays out five challenges for communities in the 1990s in responding to the HIV epidemic. These challenges include: (1) community organizing; (2) risk taking; (3) embracing conflict; (4) building partnerships; and (5) building leadership for coalitions.

COMMUNITY ORGANIZING

The history of HIV prevention in San Francisco started with organizing in the gay community. Incorporated in 1982 as the Bay Area's first community-based AIDS organization, the San Francisco AIDS Foundation, as it soon became known, evolved from an earlier coalition of gay activists and physicians who had been alarmed by a rare cancer, Kaposi's sarcoma, that appeared to be striking clusters of gay men. These men and women—some with training in health education, most without—collected the sketchy data available, established an information hotline and began printing brochures directed at gay men. The Foundation's first information sheet consisted of the "10 Facts About AIDS." Nearly ten years later, the Foundation maintains a 48-volume AIDS encyclopedia for use by staff and volunteers.

Over time, what happened was relatively simple: a community educated itself to save lives. As funding became available, prevention campaigns were mounted, using billboards and newspapers and brochures. Community forums were organized. Condoms were distributed in bars and on street corners. The rate of new HIV infections among gay men in San Francisco dropped from 18 percent in 1982-84 to 5 percent during the first half of 1985 and to less than 3 percent in 1989. Similarly, sharp declines in cases of rectal gonorrhea and syphilis among gay men also have been documented.

Likewise, in 1986 San Francisco's Black and Hispanic communities began organizing to educate their own members about the risk of HIV infection. Examples of the culturally relevant education tools that have come from within these communities include a Hispanic soap opera produced by the Latino AIDS Project and an AIDS rap contest for Black high school students conducted by the Bayview-Hunters Point Foundation, a Black community service agency, and the Department of Public Health. These efforts, conceptualized and implemented by members of the affected communities, have brought the messages of risk and risk reduction to individuals once convinced AIDS was a disease of gay White men alone.

RISK TAKING

AIDS educators in all communities who charge forward with prevention campaigns find themselves quickly attacked for violating prevailing social norms relating to homosexuality in particular, sex in general, and the treatment of drug users. Norms must be challenged to get appropriate prevention messages into the hands of the people who need them. Often this entails taking risks and facing challenges.

When those social norms are codified in government regulations, the stakes become even higher. For example, the Office of AIDS of the California Department of Health Services, until changes were made in 1989, banned the use of the words "condom" and "bleach" and "anal sex" in any material paid for with its monies. This state-engineered censorship forced HIV program administrators in smaller counties throughout California—programs funded almost entirely through state contracts—either to forego disseminating certain messages or to begin private fundraising to buy or to produce brochures using the accepted slang of their audiences.

Even in San Francisco, there has been resistance by local government to some innovations in marketing risk reduction messages. A condom poster aimed specifically at gay men and depicting a single male nude was opposed by the city's health department as likely to incite a conservative backlash in the city. After two years in circulation, no such backlash has occurred. Rather the poster, through its ongoing distribution in gay communities around the globe, has helped keep the condom message current for gay men in many nations.

Meanwhile, a San Francisco campaign to reach injection drug users was another education effort surrounded by controversy. Known as the "Bleachman" campaign, this prevention effort was designed to get needle users to clean their shooting apparatus with bleach. Some high level public officials and community leaders saw the campaign as promoting drug use. Data from precampaign focus group testing of the material did not support this fear, however. Scientific sampling after the campaign verified Bleachman's success in selling the bleach message to the targeted audiences. Eighty-nine percent of persons interviewed in a survey said they had heard of Bleachman; 88 percent claimed they were now more likely to flush their needles with bleach.

In both these campaigns, battles had to be fought to get life-saving messages into production and out to constituents. The fight over the propriety of the condom poster stretched over several meetings involving city funders and San Francisco AIDS Foundation staff. After little progress, the city's top health official was confronted and told the poster was crucial to prevention efforts among San Francisco's gay men. The Foundation was set on publishing it without his approval. The official relented. And the lesson is clear: AIDS educators must be prepared to push social norms and community leaders to new limits in order to stop the spread of HIV infection.

EMBRACING CONFLICT

San Francisco AIDS Foundation staff also have learned to embrace public controversies as powerful prevention tools. For instance, the first time safe sex messages blanketed the headlines and airwaves in San Francisco came during the 1984 fight to close the city's bathhouses. For two years, AIDS activists had been struggling to get their prevention messages into the mainstream media and were in the midst of planning their latest attempt, an AIDS awareness week, when the bathhouse controversy erupted.

In short time, San Franciscans got a lively education on the sexual transmission of AIDS as the bathhouse debate aired night after night on local news broadcasts. In the end, public conflict over HIV prevention strategies was used to garner the media spotlight to lend support to educational efforts.

BUILDING PARTNERSHIPS

San Franciscans also have found that it is crucial to have partnerships with powerful and influential individuals and institutions in place when controversies erupt. A particularly productive media partnership for the San Francisco AIDS Foundation grew out of an early conflict over the question of risk of HIV infection to heterosexuals. In an editorial, a San Francisco newspaper questioned the reliability of a Foundation-sponsored survey of the sexual practices of the city's single heterosexuals. The Foundation had concluded that a major portion of the survey respondents were putting themselves at risk for HIV infection through unprotected sex with multiple partners. The editorial charged the conclusion was not true, that it was a manipulation by "homosexual activists" to gain sympathy for their cause.

The Foundation demanded a meeting with the editorial board and presented its evidence. Having been persuaded, the newspaper agreed to run stories highlighting HIV infection risks for heterosexuals. Three months later, the U.S. Surgeon General released his first report on AIDS, which made the same assertions as the Foundation's earlier report. The myth of AIDS as a "gay disease" was finally being shattered, and the Foundation had formed a productive relationship with a newspaper staff that continues to the present.

136

A second arena for partnerships, one that can attract both dollars and credibility for groundbreaking prevention efforts, is the business community. In San Francisco, initial partnerships with a corporate coalition provided entree to the San Francisco AIDS Foundation for HIV education programs in the workplace. There was need both for fear reduction among coworkers of persons diagnosed with AIDS and for general prevention messages. This partnership produced a print and video instructional package, *An Epidemic of Fear: AIDS in the Workplace*, that has been sold to more than 2,000 corporations nationwide. Purchasers have included United Airlines, Apple Computer, GTE Sprint and the Hewlett-Packard Company.

Because of the good working relationships forged in this initial joint venture, business leaders began to give monies to varied prevention projects of the Foundation. These business leaders formed a corporate advisory body to the Foundation in 1988. Among its other contributions, the group was able to generate significant "downtown" dollars to oppose and defeat the counterproductive AIDS reporting initiatives on the 1988 California state ballot—the first time most of these enterprises had given time or funds to any AIDS-related political campaign.

None of the partnerships described here, none of the initial organizing and little of the ongoing HIV prevention work goes easily. Passions run high. Strongly held values clash. Taking power to save lives often requires bitter battles. Success only seems to lead to the next challenge.

BUILDING LEADERSHIP FOR COALITIONS

Broad-based leadership in overcoming these challenges or barriers is essential. In San Francisco, the Department of Public Health, in designing its initial responses to the emerging epidemic, sought to provide leadership in building coalitions with organizations, first in the gay community and later in the ethnic communities. With the backing of the city's elected officials and with its established paths to local, state and federal public health dollars, the health department was best equipped to forge and coordinate the necessary coalitions.

In locales where public health agencies have failed to take the lead in the AIDS fight, organizing is more difficult. Instead of attempted coordination among community-based groups, competition for turf and money is the rule. Where public health leadership is lacking, it is important that community organizers lobby their elected leaders— be they mayors, city council members or county supervisors—to facilitate their health departments becoming local leaders in the fight against HIV disease and to assist government entities in forming partnerships with community-based organizations.

Building effective coalitions also requires confronting racism, homophobia and sexism. In San Francisco, this has meant White gay men tackling their own racism, members of ethnic groups looking at their rejection of homosexuality, and all groups and communities seeking to understand the special problems of women with HIV infection. Communities also have had to come to terms with substance use among their own, as more drug treatment options are called for, in addition to the distribution of needles and bleach, to save drug users' lives.

As the stereotypes and prejudices that keep groups apart are overcome, coalitions will form across affected communities to build a stronger political voice for the resources needed in HIV prevention campaigns. Those who control the funds, be they government, business or private donors, are better approached with a unified and broad-based appeal for help.

CONCLUSION

In San Francisco, HIV prevention started with a small band of storefront activists and concerned doctors. We built our power from the ground up. We've taken on allies where we could find them. We've struggled to be ever more inclusive, to break through barriers and bigotry as we encountered them. We have built leadership, we have built power, we have built hope, we have built community. This is not to say that all is done. Despite our successes, we still face the painful struggle of building these coalitions as new issues emerge and as dollars continue to be in short supply.

As a result, lifestyles are being changed. The initial payoff has been radically altered sexual habits among gay men. The concurrent focus on the injection drug culture has produced evidence of preventing a second wave of HIV infections among needle users. The more profound result has been the development of a community-based HIV prevention model that allows individuals and groups to define their own problems and seek their own solutions.

Our aim in this book has been to link arms with people in every community of the United States to stop this plague of the late twentieth century. It has also been to highlight the crucial difference that individuals and communities can make in shaping the future course of this disease. We *can* end this epidemic—person by person, community by community.

Notes

CHAPTER 1
A Modern Epidemic Emerges: History and Context

1. Centers for Disease Control. 1990. *HIV/AIDS Surveillance Report* (January).

Centers for Disease Control. 1987. Human immunodeficiency virus infection in the United States: A review of current knowledge. *Morbidity and Mortality Weekly Report* 36 (Suppl S-6): 1-19.

Heyward, W.L. and Curran, J.W. 1988. The epidemiology of AIDS in the United States. *Scientific American* (October): 72-78.

2. Centers for Disease Control. 1989. Update: Acquired immunodeficiency syndrome—United States, 1981-1988. *Morbidity and Mortality Weekly Report* 38:234.

Centers for Disease Control. *HIV/AIDS Surveillance Report (January).*

3. Nakajima, H. 1990. World Health Organization Statement to WHO Global Programme on AIDS, Geneva, April 26.

Mann, J.M. and Chin, J. 1988. AIDS: A global perspective. *New England Journal of Medicine* 319:302-303.

4. Centers for Disease Control. 1981. Pneumocystis pneumonia—Los Angeles. *Morbidity and Mortality Weekly Report* 30:250-252.

Centers for Disease Control. 1981. Kaposi's sarcoma and Pneumocystis pneumonia among homosexual men—New York City and California. *Morbidity and Mortality Weekly Report* 30:305-308.

5. Jaffe, H.W., Bregman, D.J. and Selik, R.M. 1983. Acquired immune deficiency syndrome in the United States: The first 1000 cases. *Journal of Infectious Diseases* 148:339-45.

6. See note 5 above.

Curran, J.W. and Morgan, M.W. 1986. Acquired immunodeficiency syndrome: The beginning, the present, the future. Foreword: Epidemiology. In *AIDS from the beginning*, ed. Cole, H.M. and Lundberg, G.D. *Journal of the American Medical Association.*

7. See note 5 above.

Amman, A.J., Cowan, M.J., Wara, D.W. et al. 1983. Acquired immunodeficiency syndrome: Possible transmission by means of blood products. *Lancet* 1:956-958.

8. See note 5 above.

9. Centers for Disease Control. 1983. Prevention of acquired immune deficiency syndrome (AIDS): Report of inter-agency recommendations. *Morbidity and Mortality Weekly Report* 32.

10. Oppenheimer, G. 1988. In the eye of the storm: The epidemiological construction of AIDS. In *AIDS: The Burdens of History*, ed. Fee, E. and Fox, D.M. Berkeley and Los Angeles: Univ. of California Press.

11. Fauci, A.S. 1983. The acquired immunodeficiency syndrome: An ever broadening clinical spectrum. *Journal of the American Medical Association* 249:2375-2376.

12. Barré-Sinoussi, F., Chermann, J.C., Rey, F. et al. 1983. Isolation of a T-lymphotropic retrovirus from a patient at risk for acquired immunodeficiency syndrome (AIDS). *Science* 220:868-871.

Gallo, R.C., Salahuddin, S.Z., Popovic, M. et al. 1984. Frequent detection and isolation of cytopathic retroviruses (HTLV-III) from patients with AIDS and at risk for AIDS. *Science* 224:500-503.

Levy, J.A., Hoffman, A.D., Kramer, S.M. et al. 1984. Isolation of lymphocytopathic retroviruses from San Francisco patients with AIDS. *Science* 225:840-842.

Brun-Vézinet, F., Rouzioux, C., Montagnier, L. et al. 1984. Prevalence of antibodies to lymphadenopathy-associated retrovirus in African patients with AIDS. *Science* 226:453-456.

13. Popovic, M., Sarngadharan, M.Q., Read, E. et al. 1984. Detection, isolation and continuous production of cytopathic retroviruses (HTLV-III) from patients with AIDS and pre-AIDS. *Science* 224:497-500.

14. McNeill, W. 1976. *Plagues and peoples.* New York: Anchor Press.

15. Kass, E. 1987. History of the specialty of infectious diseases in the United

States. *Annals of Internal Medicine* 106:745-756.

16. See note 14 above.

Zahradnik, J.M. and Cherry, J.D. 1987. Influenza viruses. Chap. 29 in *Textbook of Pediatric Infectious Diseases*, Vol. 2, ed. Feigin, R.D. and Cherry, J.D. Philadelphia: W.B. Saunders.

17. Brandt, A.M. 1988. The syphilis epidemic and its relation to AIDS. *Science* 239:375-380.

18. See note 17 above.

Brandt, A.M. 1988. AIDS in historical perspective: Four lessons from the history of sexually transmitted diseases. *American Journal of Public Health* 78:367-371.

19. Brandt, A.M. 1985. *No magic bullet.* New York: Oxford Univ. Press.

20. See note 17 above.

21. Dowling, H.F. 1977. *Fighting infection: Conquests of the twentieth century.* Cambridge, MA: Harvard Univ. Press.

22. Brandt, AIDS in historical perspective.

23. See note 17 above.

24. Cutler, J.C. and Arnold, R.C. 1988. Venereal disease control by health departments in the past: Lessons for the present. *American Journal of Public Health* 78:372-376.

25. Centers for Disease Control. 1989. Congenital syphilis—New York City, 1986-1988. *Morbidity and Mortality Weekly Report* 38:825-829.

DesJarlais, D.C. and Friedman, S.R. 1988. Intravenous cocaine, crack and HIV infection. *Journal of the American Medical Association* 259:1945-1946.

26. Centers for Disease Control. 1989. Summary of notifiable diseases United States, 1988. *Morbidity and Mortality Weekly Report* 37(54): 51.

27. See note 17 above.

Cutler and Arnold, Venereal disease control.

28. Dowling, *Fighting infection.*

Sandritter, W. and Thomas, C. 1977. *Macropathology.* New York: Schattauer Verl.

29. Hulley, S.B. 1988. Principles of preventive medicine. Chap. 10 in *Cecil Textbook of Medicine*, ed. Wyngaarden, J.B. and Smith, L.H. Philadelphia: W.B. Saunders.

30. Kaslow, R.A. and Francis, D.P. 1989. Epidemiology: General considerations. Chap. 7 in *The epidemiology of AIDS*, ed. Kaslow, R.A. and Francis, D.P. New York: Oxford Univ. Press.

Essex, M. 1989. The origin of human retroviruses. Presented at the 5th International Conference on AIDS, Montreal.

31. Clavel, F., Guétard, D., Brun-Vézinet, F. et al. 1986. Isolation of a new human retrovirus from West African patients with AIDS. *Science* 233:343-346.

Centers for Disease Control. 1989. Update: HIV-2 infection—United States. *Morbidity and Mortality Weekly Report* 38:572-574; 579-580.

32. Fultz, P. 1989. The biology of human immunodeficiency viruses. Chap. 1 in *The epidemiology of AIDS*, ed. Kaslow, R.A. and Francis, D.P. New York: Oxford Univ. Press.

Levy, J. 1989. Human immunodeficiency viruses and the pathogenesis of AIDS. *Journal of the American Medical Association* 261:2997-3006.

Levy, J.A., Cheng-Mayer, C., Walker, C. et al. 1989. Viral and host factors influencing the progression to AIDS. Presented at the 5th International Conference on AIDS, Montreal.

33. Ho, D.D., Mongdil, T. and Alain, M. 1989. Quantitation of human immunodeficiency virus type 1 in the blood of infected persons. *New England Journal of Medicine* 321:1621-1625.

Coombs, R.W., Collier, A.C., Allain, J.P. et al. 1989. Plasma viremia in human immunodeficiency virus infection. *New England Journal of Medicine* 321:1626-1631.

34. Fultz, Biology of human immunodeficiency viruses.

Levy, Human immunodeficiency viruses.

35. Fultz, Biology of human immunodeficiency viruses.

36. Saag, M.S., Hahn, B.H., Gibbons, J. et al. 1988. Extensive variation of human immunodeficiency virus in vivo. *Nature* 334:440-444.

Fenjö, E.M., Albert, J., Morfeldt-Månson L. et al. 1989. Replication capacity of sequential virus isolates from HIV-1 infected subjects and relationship to clinical progression. Presented at the 5th International Conference on AIDS, Montreal.

37. Levy et al., Viral and host factors.

Cheng-Mayer, C., Seto, D., Tateno, M. et al. 1988. Biologic features of HIV-1 that correlate with virulence in the host. *Science* 240:80-82.

38. Fenjö et al., Replication capacity.

Cheng-Mayer et al., Biologic features of HIV-1.

39. Levy, J.A., Evans, L., Cheng-Mayer, C. et al. 1987. Biologic and molecular properties of the AIDS-associated retrovirus that affect antiviral therapy. *Annales de l'Institut de Pasteur—Virology* 138:101-111.

40. Levy, Human immunodeficiency viruses.

Bolognesi, D. 1989. Prospects for prevention of and early intervention against HIV. *Journal of the American Medical Association* 261:3007-3013.

41. Bolognesi, Prospects for prevention.

42. Lifson, A.R., Rutherford, G.W. and Jaffe, H.W. 1988. The natural history of human immunodeficiency virus infection. *Journal of Infectious Diseases* 158:1360-1367.

Ranki, A., Valle, S.L., Krohn, M. et al. 1987. Long latency precedes overt seroconversion in sexually transmitted human immunodeficiency virus infection. *Lancet* 2:589-593.

Imagawa, D.T., Lee, M.H., Wolinsky, S.M. et al. 1989. Human immunodeficiency virus type 1 infection in homosexual men who remain seronegative for prolonged periods. *New England Journal of Medicine* 320:1458-1462.

Haseltine, W.A. 1989. Silent HIV infection. Editorial review. *New England Journal of Medicine* 320:1487-1489.

Wolinsky, S.M., Rinaldo, C.R., Kwok, S. et al. 1989. Human immunodeficiency virus type 1 (HIV-1) infection a median of 18 months before a diagnostic Western Blot. *Annals of Internal Medicine* 111:961-972.

43. See note 33 above.

44. Jackson, J.B. and Balfour, H.H. 1988. Practical diagnostic testing for human immunodeficiency virus. *Clinical Microbiology Review* 1:124-138.

Phair, J.P. and Wolinsky, S. 1989. Diagnosis of infection with the human immunodeficiency virus. *Journal of Infectious Diseases* 159:320-323.

45. Levy et al., Viral and host factors.

Ho, D.D., Byington, R.E., Schooley, R.T. et al. 1985. Infrequency of isolation of HTLV-III virus from saliva in AIDS. *New England Journal of Medicine* 313:1606.

46. Levy et al., Viral and host factors.

Kreiss, J.K., Coombs, R., Plummer, F. et al. 1989. Isolation of human immunodeficiency virus from genital ulcers in Nairobi prostitutes. *Journal of Infectious Diseases* 160:380-384.

47. Centers for Disease Control. 1989. Interpretation and use of the Western blot assay for serodiagnosis of human immunodeficiency virus type 1 infection. *Morbidity and Mortality Weekly Report* 38 (Suppl S-7).

48. Lo, B., Steinbrook, R.L., Cooke, M. et al. 1989. Voluntary screening for human immunodeficiency virus (HIV) infection. *Annals of Internal Medicine* 110:727-733.

Burke, D.S., Brundage, J.F., Redfield, R.R. et al. 1988. Measurement of false positive rate in a screening program for human immunodeficiency virus infections. *New England Journal of Medicine* 319:961-964.

49. Centers for Disease Control. 1987. Revision of the Centers for Disease Control surveillance case definition for acquired immunodeficiency syndrome. *Morbidity and Mortality Weekly Report* 36 (Suppl S-1).

50. Conway, G.A., Colby-Niemeyer, B., Pursley, C. et al. 1989. Underreporting of AIDS cases in South Carolina, 1986 and 1987. *Journal of the American Medical Association* 262:2859-2863.

51. Stoneburner, R.L., DesJarlais, D.C., Benezra, D. et al. 1988. A larger spectrum of severe HIV-1 related disease in intravenous drug users. *Science* 242:916-919.

Centers for Disease Control. 1988. Increase in pneumonia mortality among young adults and the HIV epidemic. *Morbidity and Mortality Weekly Report* 37:593-596.

Selwyn, P.A., Hartel, D., Wasserman, W. et al. 1989. Impact of the AIDS epidemic on morbidity and mortality among intravenous drug users in a New York City methadone maintenance program. *American Journal of Public Health* 79:1358-1362.

52. Centers for Disease Control. 1988. AIDS and human immunodeficiency virus infection in the United States: 1988 update. *Morbidity and Mortality Weekly Report* 38(Suppl S-4).

53. Selwyn et al., Impact of AIDS epidemic.

54. Lifson et al., Natural history.

55. See note 52 above.

Anderson, R.M. and Medley, G.F. Epidemiology of HIV infection and AIDS: Incubation and infectious periods, survival and vertical transmission. *AIDS* 2 (Suppl): 57-63.

Moss, A.R. and Bacchetti, P. 1989. Natural history of HIV infection. Editorial review. *AIDS* 3:56-61.

Lemp, G.F., Payne, S.F., Rutherford, G.W. et al. 1990. Projections of AIDS morbidity and mortality in San Francisco. *Journal of the American Medical Association* 263:1497-1501.

56. Curran, J.W., Jaffe, H.W., Hardy, A.M. et al. 1988. Epidemiology of HIV infection and AIDS in the United States. *Science* 239:610-616.

Lui, K.J., Darrow, W.W. and Rutherford, G.W. 1988. A model-based estimate of the mean incubation period for AIDS in homosexual men. *Science* 240:1333-1335.

57. Marx, J. 1989. Wider use of AIDS drug advocated. *Science* 245:811.

Lemp, G.F., Payne, S.F., Neal, D. et al. 1990. Survival trends for patients with AIDS. *Journal of the American Medical Association* 263:402-406.

58. Anderson and Medley, Epidemiology of HIV infection and AIDS.

59. Lemp et al., Survival trends.

60. Krasinski, K., Borkowsky, W., Holzman, R.S. et al. 1989. Prognosis of human immunodeficiency virus infection in children and adolescents. *Pediatric Infectious Disease Journal* 8:216-220.

61. Scott, G.B., Hutto, C., Makuch, R.W. et al. 1989. Survival in children with perinatally acquired human immunodeficiency virus type 1 infection. *New England Journal of Medicine* 321:1791-1796.

CHAPTER 2
Patterns of the Epidemic and Public Health Implications

1. Hulley, S. and Hearst, N. 1989. The worldwide epidemiology and prevention of AIDS. In *Primary prevention of AIDS*, ed. Mays, V., Alber, G. and Schneider, S. Newbury Park, CA: Sage Publications.

Mann, J. and Chin, J. 1988. AIDS: A global perspective. *New England Journal of Medicine* 319:302-303.

2. Centers for Disease Control. 1984. *AIDS Weekly Surveillance Report* (July 30).

Centers for Disease Control. 1990. *HIV/AIDS Surveillance Report* (January).

3. Centers for Disease Control. 1990. *HIV/AIDS Surveillance Report* (Janu-

ary).

4. See note 3 above.

5. Manoff, S., Gayle, H., Mays, M. et al. 1989. Acquired immunodeficiency syndrome in adolescents: Epidemiology, prevention and public health issues. *Pediatric Infectious Disease Journal* 8:309-314.

6. See note 3 above.

Centers for Disease Control. 1989. Update: Acquired immunodeficiency syndrome—United States, 1981-1988. *Morbidity and Mortality Weekly Report* 38(14).

Centers for Disease Control. 1989. First 100,000 cases of acquired immunodeficiency syndrome—United States. *Morbidity and Mortality Weekly Report* 38(32).

7. See note 3 above.

Centers for Disease Control. 1989. AIDS and human immunodeficiency virus infection in the United States: 1988 update. *Morbidity and Mortality Weekly Report* 38 (Suppl S-4).

8. Haverkos, H., Edelman, R. et al. 1988. The epidemiology of acquired immunodeficiency syndrome among heterosexuals. *Journal of the American Medical Association* 260:1922-1929.

9. Centers for Disease Control. 1990. Update: Acquired immunodeficiency syndrome—United States, 1989. *Morbidity and Mortality Weekly Report* 39(5).

10. Novick, L., Berns, D., Stricof, R. et al. 1989. HIV seroprevalence in newborns in New York State. *Journal of the American Medical Association* 261:1745-1750.

Capell, F., Nordaunt, V., Vugia, D. et al. 1989. Distribution of HIV infection among childbearing women in California: Results from the first wave of unlinked neonatal HIV screening. Presented at the 5th National Pediatric AIDS Conference, Los Angeles.

11. Centers for Disease Control. AIDS and human immunodeficiency virus infection in the United States: 1988 update.

12. Fullilove, R., Fullilove, M., Bowser, B. et al. 1990. Risk of sexually transmitted disease among Black adolescent crack users in Oakland and San Francisco, Calif. *Journal of the American Medical Association* 263:851-855.

13. See note 5 above.

14. Centers for Disease Control. 1989. HIV reporting—United States. *Morbidity and Mortality Weekly Report* 38(28).

15. See note 11 above.

16. Palca, J. 1989. Is the AIDS epidemic slowing? *Science* 246:1560.

17. See note 11 above.

Winkelstein, W., Lyman, D., Padian, N. et al. 1987. Sexual practices and risk of infection by the human immunodeficiency virus: The San Francisco men's health study. *Journal of the American Medical Association* 257:321-325.

Hessol, N., O'Malley, P., Lifson, A. et al. 1989. Incidence and prevalence of HIV infection among homosexual and bisexual men, 1978-1988. Presented at the 5th International Conference on AIDS, Montreal.

18. Quinn, T., Glassner, D., Cannon, R. et al. 1988. Human immunodeficiency virus infection among patients attending clinics for sexually transmitted diseases. *New England Journal of Medicine* 318:197-202.

Centers for Disease Control. 1987. Human immunodeficiency virus infection in the United States: A review of current knowledge. *Morbidity and Mortality Weekly Report* 36(Suppl S-6).

19. Hessol et al., Incidence and prevalence of HIV infection.

Winkelstein, W., Samuel, M., Padian, N. et al. 1987. The San Francisco men's health study: III (1982-86). *American Journal of Public Health* 76:685-689.

Winkelstein, W., Wiley, J., Padian, N. et al. 1988. The San Francisco men's health study: Continued decline in HIV seroconversion rates among homosexual/bisexual men. *American Journal of Public Health* 78:1472-1474.

20. Centers for Disease Control. Human immunodeficiency virus infection in the United States: A review of current knowledge.

DesJarlais, D., Friedman, S., Novick, D. et al. 1989. HIV-1 infection among intravenous drug users in Manhattan, New York City, from 1977 through 1987. *Journal of the American Medical Association* 261:1008-1012.

21. See note 11 above.

Centers for Disease Control. Human immunodeficiency virus in the United States: A review of current knowledge.

Watters, J., Lewis, D., Cheng, Y.T. et al. 1988. Drug-use profile, risk participation and HIV exposure among intravenous drug users in San Francisco. Presented at the 4th International Conference on AIDS, Stockholm.

22. DesJarlais, D., Friedman, S. and Stoneburner, R. 1988. HIV infection and intravenous drug use: Critical issues in transmission dynamics, infection outcomes, and prevention. *Reviews of Infectious Diseases* 10:151-158.

DesJarlais, D. and Friedman, S. 1990. Shooting galleries and AIDS: Infection probabilities and tough policies. *American Journal of Public Health* 80:142-144.

Chitwood, D., McCoy, C., Inciardi. D. et al. 1990. HIV seropositivity of needles from shooting galleries in South Florida. *American Journal of Public Health* 80:150-152.

23. Lange, R., Snyder, F., Lozovsky, D. et al. 1988. Geographic distribution of human immunodeficiency markers in parenteral drug abusers. *American Journal of Public Health* 78:443-446.

24. Moss, A. 1987. AIDS and intravenous drug use: The real heterosexual epidemic. *British Medical Journal* 294:389-390.

25. See note 8 above.

26. See note 11 above.

27. Hearst, N. and Hulley, S. 1988. Preventing the heterosexual spread of AIDS: Are we giving our patients the best advice? *Journal of the American Medical Association* 259:2428-2432.

28. See note 11 above.

29. See note 11 above.

30. Centers for Disease Control, Human immunodeficiency virus in the United States: A review of current knowledge.

31. Hulley and Hearst, Worldwide epidemiology.

See note 11 above.

Cumming, P., Wallace, E., Schorr, J. et al. 1989. Exposure of patients to human immunodeficiency virus through the transfusion of blood components that test antibody-negative. *New England Journal of Medicine* 321:941-946.

32. Hulley and Hearst, Worldwide epidemiology.

See note 11 above.

See note 27 above.

33. See note 11 above.

See note 10 above.

Hoff, R., Berardi, V. and Weiblen, B. 1988. Seroprevalence of human immunodeficiency virus among childbearing women. *New England Journal of Medicine* 318:525-530.

Altman, R., Grant, C., Brandon, D. et al. 1989. Statewide HIV-1 serologic survey of newborns with resultant changes in screening and delivery system policy. Presented at the 5th International Conference on AIDS, Montreal.

Papaioannou, M., George, R., Haimon, H. et al. 1989. National surveys of HIV seroprevalence in women delivering live children in the United States. Presented at the 5th International Conference on AIDS, Montreal.

34. Novick et al., HIV seroprevalence in newborns.

Landesman, S., Minkoff, H., Holman, S. et al. 1987. Serosurvey of human immunodeficiency virus in parturients. *Journal of the American Medical Association* 258:2701-2703.

Krasinski, K., Borkovsky, W., Bebenroth, D. et al. 1988. Failure of voluntary testing for human immunodeficiency virus to identify infected parturient women in a high risk population. *New England Journal of Medicine* 318:185.

35. Capell et al., Distribution of HIV infection.

36. Novick et al., HIV seroprevalence in newborns.

37. See note 30 above.

Chaisson, R., Osmond, D., Moss, A. et al. 1987. HIV, bleach and needle sharing. *Lancet* 1:1430.

38. See note 11 above.

39. Kolata, G. 1989. AIDS is spreading in teen-agers, a new trend alarming to experts. *New York Times*, October 8.

40. See note 11 above.

Centers for Disease Control. 1988. HIV-related beliefs, knowledge and behaviors among high school students. *Morbidity and Mortality Weekly Report* 37.

Hein, K. 1989. Commentary on adolescent acquired immunodeficiency syndrome: The next wave of the human immunodeficiency virus epidemic? *Journal of Pediatrics* 114:144-149.

41. Centers for Disease Control. HIV-related beliefs, knowledge and behav-

iors among high-school students.

Kegeles, S., Adler, N. and Irwin, C. 1988. Sexually active adolescents and condoms: Changes over one year in knowledge, attitudes and use. *American Journal of Public Health* 78:460-461.

42. Gail, M.H. and Brookmeyer, R. 1988. Methods for projecting course of acquired immunodeficiency syndrome epidemic. *Journal of the National Cancer Institute* 80:900-911.

43. Marx, J. 1989. Wider use of AIDS drug advocated. *Science* 245:811.

Lemp, G., Payne, S., Neal, D. et al. 1990. Survival trends for patients with AIDS. *Journal of the American Medical Association* 263:402-406.

44. Lemp, G., Payne, S., Rutherford, G. et al. 1988. Projections of AIDS morbidity and mortality in San Francisco using epidemic models. Presented at the 4th International Conference on AIDS, Stockholm.

45. Fultz, P. 1989. The biology of human immunodeficiency viruses. In *The epidemiology of AIDS*, ed. Kaslow, R. and Francis, D. New York: Oxford Univ. Press.

46. Winkelstein et al., Sexual practices.

Polk, B., Fox, R., Brookmeyer, R. et al. 1987. Predictors of the acquired immunodeficiency syndrome developing in a cohort of seropositive homosexual men. *New England Journal of Medicine* 316:61-66.

Winkelstein, W., Padian, N., Rutherford, G. et al. 1989. Homosexual men. In *The epidemiology of AIDS*, ed. Kaslow, R. and Francis, D. et al. New York: Oxford Univ. Press.

47. Winkelstein et al., Homosexual men.

48. Holmberg, S., Horsburgh, C., Ward, J. et al. 1989. Biologic factors in the sexual transmission of human immunodeficiency virus. *Journal of Infectious Diseases* 160:116-125.

49. See note 48 above.

Padian, N. 1987. Heterosexual transmission of acquired immunodeficiency syndrome: International perspectives and national projections. *Reviews of Infectious Diseases* 9:947-991.

50. Goedert, J., Eyster, M., Biggar, R. et al. 1988. Heterosexual transmission of human immunodeficiency virus: Association with severe depletion of T-helper lymphocytes in men with hemophilia. *AIDS Research and Human Retroviruses* 3:355-36.

Osmond, D., Bacchetti, P., Chaisson, R. et al. 1988. Time of exposure and risk of HIV infection in homosexual partners of men with AIDS. *American Journal of Public Health* 78:944-948.

51. Cameron, D., D'Costa, L., Maitha, G.M. et al. 1989. Female to male transmission of human immunodeficiency virus type 1: Risk factors for seroconversion in men. *Lancet* 2:403-407.

Latif, A., Katzenstein, D., Bassett, M. et al. 1989. Genital ulcers and transmission of HIV among couples in Zimbabwe. *AIDS* 3:519-523.

52. See note 24 above.

53. Padian, N., Marquis, L. and Francis, D. 1987. Male-to-female transmission of human immunodeficiency virus. *Journal of the American Medical Association* 258:788-790.

Peterman, T., Stoneburner, R., Allen, J. et al. 1988. Risk of human immunodeficiency virus transmission from heterosexual adults with transfusion-associated infections. *Journal of the American Medical Association* 259:55-58.

54. See note 48 above.

55. Peterman et al., Risk of human immunodeficiency virus transmission.

56. See note 27 above.

57. See note 27 above.

58. Levy, J. 1989. Human immunodeficiency viruses and the pathogenesis of AIDS. *Journal of the American Medical Association* 261:2997-3006.

59. Stewart, G., Tyler, J., Cunningham, A. et al. 1985. Transmission of human T-cell lymphotropic virus type III (HTLV-III) by artificial insemination by donor. *Lancet* 2:581-584.

60. Cameron et al., Female to male transmission.

Piot, P., Plummer, F., Mhalu, F. et al. 1988. AIDS: An international perspective. *Science* 239:573-579.

Greenblatt, R., Lukehart, S., Plummer, F. et al. 1988. Genital ulceration as a risk factor for human immunodeficiency virus infection. *AIDS* 2:47-50.

Marx, J. 1989. Circumcision may protect against the AIDS virus. *Science* 245:470-471.

61. Kreiss, J., Coombs, R., Plummer, F. et al. 1989. Isolation of human immunodeficiency virus from genital ulcers in Nairobi prostitutes. *Journal of Infectious Diseases* 160:380-384.

62. See note 58 above.

63. Quinn et al., Human immunodeficiency virus infection.

64. Office of AIDS, State of California Department of Health Services. 1989. HIV transmission via oral sex. *California AIDS Update* 2:106.

65. Curran, J., Jaffe, H., Hardy, A. et al. 1988. Epidemiology of HIV infection and AIDS in the United States. *Science* 239:610-616.

66. Cumming et al., Exposure of patients.

67. Ward, J., Holmberg, S., Allen, J. et al. 1988. Transmission of human immunodeficiency virus (HIV) by blood transfusions screened as negative for HIV antibodies. *New England Journal of Medicine* 318:473-478.

Kleinman, S. and Secord, K. 1988. Risk of human immunodeficiency virus (HIV) transmission by anti-HIV negative blood. Estimates using lookback methodology. *Transfusion* 28:499-501.

Leitman, S., Klein, H., Melpolder, J. et al. 1989. Clinical implications of positive tests for antibodies to human immunodeficiency virus type 1 in asymptomatic blood donors. *New England Journal of Medicine* 321:917-924.

68. Leitman et al., Clinical implications.

69. Peterman et al., Risk of human immunodeficiency virus transmission.

70. Schimpf, K., Brackman, H., Kreuz, W. et al. 1989. Absence of anti-human immunodeficiency virus type 1 and 2 seroconversion after the treatment of hemophilia H or von Willebrand's disease with pasteurized factor VIII concentrate. *New England Journal of Medicine* 321:1148-1152.

Menitove, J. 1989. The decreasing risk of transfusion-associated AIDS. *New England Journal of Medicine* 321:966-968.

71. Chitwood et al., HIV seropositivity of needles.

72. See note 23 above.

Chaisson, R., Moss, A. and Onishi, R. 1987. Human immunodeficiency virus infection in heterosexual intravenous drug users in San Francisco. *American Journal of Public Health* 77:169-171.

73. Gerberding, J. and Bryant-Le Blanc, C. 1987. Risk of transmitting the human immunodeficiency virus, cytomegalovirus and hepatitis B virus to health care workers exposed to patients with AIDS and AIDS-related conditions. *Journal of Infectious Diseases* 156:1-8.

Henderson, D. and Gerberding, J. 1989. Prophylactic zidovudine after occupational exposure to the human immunodeficiency virus: An interim analysis. *Journal of Infectious Diseases* 160:321-327.

74. Joncas, J., Delage, G., Chad, Z. et al. 1983. Acquired (or congenital) immunodeficiency syndrome in infants born to Haitian mothers. *New England Journal of Medicine* 308:842.

Sprecher, S., Soumenkoff, G., Puissant, F. et al. 1986. Vertical transmission of HIV in 15-week fetus. *Lancet* 2:288-289.

Jovaisas, E., Koch, M., Schäfer, A. et al. 1985. LAV/HTLV-III in 20-week fetus. *Lancet* 2:1129.

Lapointe, N., Michaud, J., Pekovic, D. et al. 1985. Transplacental transmission of HTLV-III virus. *New England Journal of Medicine* 312:1325-1326.

75. Maury, W., Potts, B., Rabson, A. 1989. HIV-1 infection of first-trimester and term human placental tissue: A possible mode of maternal-fetal transmission. *Journal of Infectious Diseases* 160:583-588.

76. Lapointe et al., Transplacental transmission.

See note 75 above.

Chiodo, F., Ricchi, E., Costigliola, P. et al. 1986. Vertical transmission of HTLV-III. *Lancet* 1:739.

Lifson, A. and Rogers, M. 1986. Vertical transmission of human immunodeficiency virus. *Lancet* 2:739.

77. Ziegler, J., Cooper, D., Johnson, R. et al. 1985. Postnatal transmission of AIDS-associated retrovirus from mother to infant. *Lancet* 1:896-898.

Thiry, L., Sprecher-Goldberger, S., Jonckeer, T. et al. 1985. Isolation of AIDS virus from cell-free breast milk of three healthy virus carriers. *Lancet* 2:891-892.

Lepage, P., van de Perre, P., Carael, M. et al. 1987. Postnatal transmission of HIV from mother to child. *Lancet* 2:400.

Rogers, M. 1987. Breast-feeding and HIV infection. *Lancet* 2:1278.

78. European Collaborative Study. 1988. Mother-to-child transmission of HIV infection. *Lancet* 2:1040-1045.

Italian Multicentre Study. Epidemiology, clinical features and prognostic factors of pediatric HIV infection. *Lancet* 2:1043-1045.

Blanche, S., Rouzioux, C., Guihard Moscato, M. et al. 1989. A prospective study of infants born to women seropositive for human immunodeficiency virus type 1. *New England Journal of Medicine* 320:1643-1689.

79. See note 65 above.

Lifson and Rogers, Vertical transmission.

Friedland, G. and Klein, R. 1987. Transmission of the human immunodeficiency virus. *New England Journal of Medicine* 317:1125-1135.

80. Lifson, A. 1988. Do alternate modes for transmission of human immunodeficiency virus exist? *Journal of the American Medical Association* 259:1353-1356.

Pape, J., Vervier, R., Jean, S. et al. 1988. Transmission and mortality of HIV infection in Haitian children. Presented at the 4th International Conference on AIDS, Stockholm.

Saah, A. 1989. HIV-1 infection in low risk populations. In *The epidemiology of AIDS*, ed. Kaslow R. and Francis, D. New York: Oxford Univ. Press.

81. See note 58 above.

Ho, D., Byington, R., Schooley, R. et al. 1985. Infrequency of isolation of HTLV-III virus from saliva in AIDS. *New England Journal of Medicine* 313:1606.

82. Friedland and Klein, Transmission of the human immunodeficiency virus. Lifson, Do alternate models for transmission exist?

83. Friedland and Klein, Transmission of the human immunodeficiency virus.

Kaslow, R. and Francis, D. 1989. Epidemiology: General considerations. In *The epidemiology of AIDS*, ed. Kaslow, R. and Francis, D. New York: Oxford Univ. Press.

84. See note 27 above.

85. See note 27 above.

86. Hulley and Hearst, Worldwide epidemiology. See note 27 above.

87. Mann and Chin, Global perspective.

88. Hearst and Hulley, Preventing the heterosexual spread of AIDS.

89. See note 27 above.

90. Hulley and Hearst, Worldwide epidemiology.

91. Leitman, S., Klein, M., Melpolder, J. et al. 1989. Clinical implications of positive tests for antibodies to human immunodeficiency virus type 1 in asymptomatic blood donors. *New England Journal of Medicine* 321:917-924.

92. Centers for Disease Control. 1990. Public Health Service statement on management of occupational exposure to human immunodeficiency virus, including considerations regarding zidovudine postexposure use. *Morbidity and Mortal-*

ity Weekly Report 39 (No. RR-1).

93. Centers for Disease Control. 1987. Recommendations for prevention of HIV transmission in health-care settings. *Morbidity and Mortality Weekly Report* 36 (Suppl S-2).

94. Shilts, R. 1987. *And the band played on.* New York: St. Martin's Press.

95. DesJarlais, D., Friedman, S. and Strug, D. 1986. AIDS among intravenous drug users: A sociocultural perspective. In *The social dimensions of AIDS: Methods and theory*, ed. Feldman, D. and Johnson, T. New York: Praeger.

96. Winkelstein et al., San Francisco men's health study: III.

Winkelstein et al., San Francisco men's health study: Continued decline.

97. Coates, T. and Greenblatt, R. 1989. Behavioral change using interventions at the community level. In *Sexually transmitted diseases*, ed. Holmes, K., Mårdh, P.A., Sparling, F. et al. New York: McGraw-Hill.

98. Puckett, S. and Bye, L. 1987. *The STOP AIDS Project: An interpersonal AIDS prevention program.* San Francisco: The STOP AIDS Project.

99. Catania, J., Coates, T., Kegeles, S. et al. 1989. Implications of the AIDS Risk Reduction Model for the gay community: The importance of perceived sexual enjoyment and help-seeking behaviors. In *Psychological approaches to the prevention of AIDS*, ed. Maysa, V., Albee S. and Schneider, S. Newbury Park, CA: Sage Publications.

100. DesJarlais, D. and Friedman, S. 1987. HIV infection among intravenous drug users: Epidemiology and risk reduction. *AIDS* 1:67-76.

101. See note 100 above.

102. Chaisson et al., HIV, bleach and needle sharing.

Watters, J. 1987. A street-based outreach model of AIDS prevention for intravenous drug users: Preliminary evaluation. *Contemporary Drug Problems* 14:411-423.

103. Guydish, J., Temoshok, L., Dilley, J. et al. In press. Evaluation of a hospital-based substance abuse intervention and referral service for HIV affected patients. *General Hospital Psychology.*

104. Sorensen, J., Guydish, J., Constantini, M. et al. 1989. Changes in needle sharing and syringe cleaning among San Francisco drug abusers. *New England Journal of Medicine* 320:807.

Moss, A., Bacchetti, P., Osmond, D. et al. 1989. Seroconversion for HIV in intravenous drug users in San Francisco. Presented at the 5th International Conference on AIDS, Montreal.

105. Moss, A., Bachetti, P., Osmond, D. et al. Seroconversion for HIV.

106. Friedman, S., DesJarlais, D., Sotheran, J. et al. 1987. AIDS and self-organization among intravenous drug users. *International Journal of Addictions* 22:201-219.

107. See note 103 above.

Peterson, J. and Marín, G. 1988. Issues in the prevention of AIDS among Black and Hispanic men. *American Psychologist* 43:871-877.

108. Freudenberg, N., Lee, J. and Silver, D. 1989. How Black and Latino community organizations respond to the AIDS epidemic: A case study in one New York City neighborhood. *AIDS Education and Prevention* 1:12-21.

109. Williams, L. 1986. AIDS risk reduction: A community health education intervention for minority high risk group members. *Health Education Quarterly* 13:407-421.

110. Stoddard, R. 1989. Paradox and paralysis: An overview of the American response to AIDS. In *Taking liberties*, ed. Carter, E. and Watney, S. London: Serpent's Tail.

111. U.S. Department of Health and Human Services. 1985. *Report of the Secretary's Task Force on Black and Minority Health*. Washington, DC: U.S. Government Printing Office.

112. Hatfield, L. 1989. Minorities lack clout despite population. *San Francisco Examiner*, August 13.

113. Altman, D. 1987. *AIDS in the mind of America*. Garden City, NY: Anchor Press.

114. See note 113 above.

115. Patton, C. 1985. *Sex and germs: The politics of AIDS*. Boston: South End Press.

CHAPTER 3
AIDS: Putting the Models to the Test

1. National Center for Health Statistics. 1987. *Report from the Bureau of the Census*. Washington, DC: U.S. Government Printing Office.

2. See note 1 above.

3. See note 1 above.

4. Higgins, M. and Thom, T. 1989. Trends in CHD in the United States. *International Journal of Epidemiology* (Suppl 1) 18 (no. 3): 58-66.

5. National Center for Health Statistics. 1982. *Blood pressure levels and hypertension in person 6-74 years: United States, 1976-1980*. Advance Data. No. 84. Washington, DC.

6. See note 4 above.

7. U.S. Department of Agriculture. 1987. *Food consumption, prices and expenditures, 1985*. Statistical bulletin No. 749. Washington, DC.

8. National Center for Health Statistics, National Heart, Lung and Blood Institute Collaborative Lipid Groups. 1987. Trends in serum cholesterol levels among U.S. adults aged 20 to 74 years. *Journal of the American Medical Association* 257:937-942.

9. See note 4 above.

10. Califano, J.A., Jr. 1979. *Healthy people: The Surgeon General's report on health promotion and disease prevention*. Stock no. 017-001-00416-2. Washington, DC: U.S. Government Printing Office.

11. U.S. Public Health Service. 1964. Smoking and health. *Report of the Advisory Committee to the Surgeon General of the Public Health Service.* PHS Publication no. 1103. U.S. Department of Health, Education and Welfare, Centers for Disease Control.

12. U.S. Department of Health and Human Services. 1989. *Reducing the health consequences of smoking: 25 years of progress. A report of the Surgeon General.* DHHS publication no. (CDC) 89-8411. Public Health Services, Centers for Disease Control, Center for Chronic Disease Prevention and Health Promotion, Office on Smoking and Health.

13. Evans, R.I. and Raines, B. 1982. Control and prevention of smoking in adolescents: A psychosocial perspective. In *Promoting adolescent health: A dialog on research and practice*, ed. Coates, T.J., Petersen, A.C. and Perry, P., 101-136. New York: Academic Press.

14. Green, L.W. 1985. Health education models. In *Behavioral health: A handbook of health enhancement and disease prevention*, ed. Matarazzo, J.D., Weiss, S.M., Herd, J.A. et al., 181-198. New York: John Wiley.

15. Janz, M., and Becker, M. 1984. The health belief model: A decade later. *Health Education Quarterly* 11:1-47.

16. Kirscht, J. 1988. The health belief model and predictions of health actions. In *Health behavior: Emerging research perspectives*, ed. Goodman, D., 27-41. New York: Plenum.

17. Chesney, M.A. In press. Health education models in AIDS prevention. In *Women and AIDS: Promoting healthy behaviors*, ed. Blumenthal, S., Eichler, A. and Weissman, G. Washington, DC: National Institute of Mental Health.

18. Caplan, R.D., Robinson, E.A.R., French, J.R.P., Caldwell, J.R. and Shinn, M. 1976. *Adhering to medical regimens: Pilot experiments in patient education and social support.* Ann Arbor: University of Michigan.

Sackett, D.L., Gibson, E.S., Taylor, D.W. et al. 1975. Randomized clinical trial of strategies for improving medication compliance in primary hypertension. *Lancet* 1:1205-1207.

19. McKusick, L., Hortsman, W. and Coates, T.J. 1985. AIDS and the sexual behavior reported by gay men in San Francisco. *American Journal of Public Health* 75:1440-1445.

20. See note 19 above.

21. Adler, N. In press. Changing risk behavior: Fear, rationality and decision making. In *Women and AIDS: Promoting healthy behaviors*, ed. Blumenthal, S., Eichler, A. and Weissman G. Washington, DC: National Institute of Mental Health.

22. See note 17 above.

23. See note 14 above.

24. Evans, R.I. 1980. Behavioral medicine: A new applied challenge to social psychologists: In *Applied social psychology annual reviews I*, ed. Bickman, L. Beverly Hills, CA: Sage Publications.

25. Weber, J., Coates, T.J. and McKusick, L. 1987. *Denial is associated with*

high risk sexual behavior among gay men in San Francisco: The AIDS Behavioral Research Project. University of California, San Francisco.

26. Jessor, R. 1985. Adolescent development and behavioral health. In *Behavioral health: A handbook of health enhancement and disease prevention*, ed. Matarazzo, J.D., Weiss, S.M., Herd, J.A. et al., 69-90. New York: John Wiley.

27. See note 26 above.

28. Azjen, I. and Fishbein, M. 1980. *Understanding attitudes and predicting social behavior.* Englewood Cliffs, NJ: Prentice-Hall.

29. Solomon, M.Z. and DeJong, W. 1986. Recent sexually transmitted disease prevention efforts and their implications for AIDS health education. *Health Education Quarterly* 13:301-316.

30. Joseph, J.G., Kessler, R.C., Wortman, C.B. et al. 1989. Are there psychological costs associated with changes in behavior to reduce AIDS risk? In *Primary Prevention of AIDS*, ed. Mays, V.M., Albee, G.W. and Schneider, S.F., 209-224. Newbury Park, CA: Sage Publications.

31. Warner, R. 1985. Communication in health care. In *Behavioral medicine: The biopsychosocial approach*, ed. Schneiderman, N. and Tapp, J.T., 45-66. Hillsdale, NJ: Lawrence Erlbaum.

32. Evans, R.I. 1985. A social inoculation strategy to deter smoking in adolescents. In *Behavioral health: A handbook of health enhancement and disease prevention*, ed. Matarazzo, J.D., Weiss, S.M., Herd, J.A. et al., 765-785. New York: John Wiley.

Evans, R.I. 1987. Health promotion: Science or ideology. Presidential Address to Division of Health Psychology, annual meeting of the American Psychological Association.

33. Gordon, N.P. and McAlister, A.L. 1982. Adolescent drinking: Issues and research. In *Promoting adolescent health: A dialog on research and practice*, ed. Coates, T.J., Petersen, A.C. and Perry, C., 201-224. New York: Academic Press.

34. Rivara, R.P. 1985. Epidemiology of childhood injuries. In *Behavioral health: A handbook of health enhancement and disease prevention*, ed. Matarazzo, J.D., Weiss, S.M., Herd, J.A. et al. New York: John Wiley.

35. Wadden, T.A. and Brownell, K.D. 1985. The development and modification of dietary practices in individuals, groups and large populations. In *Behavioral health: A handbook of health enhancement and disease prevention*, ed. Matarazzo, J.D., Weiss, S.M., Herd, J.A. et al., 603-631. New York: John Wiley.

36. Kegeles, S.S. and Lund, A.K. 1985. Adolescents' acceptance of caries-preventive procedures. In *Behavioral health: A handbook of health enhancement and disease prevention*, ed. Matarazzo, J.D., Weiss, S.M., Herd, J.A. et al., 895-909. New York: John Wiley.

37. Bandura, A. 1990. Perceived self-efficacy in the exercise of control over AIDS infection. *Evaluation and program planning* 13:9-17.

38. Brod, M.I. and Hall, S.M. 1984. Joiners and non-joiners in smoking treatment: A comparison of psychosocial variables. *Addictive Behaviors* 9:217-221.

39. See note 37 above, p. 137.
40. Morin, S.F., Charles, K., Coates, T.J. and McKusick, L. 1987. *AIDS: Helping patients to reduce risk.* University of California, San Francisco.
41. See note 40 above.
42. See note 37 above, p. 137.
43. Farquhar, J.W., Fortmann, S.P., Maccoby, N. et al. 1985. The Stanford Five City Project: An Overview (1985). In *Behavioral health: A handbook of health enhancement and disease prevention*, ed. Matarazzo, J.D., Weiss, S.M., Herd, J.A. et al., 1154-1165. New York: John Wiley.

Blackburn, H., Luepker, R.W., Kline, F.G. et al. 1985. The Minnesota Heart Health Program: A research and demonstration project in cardiovascular disease prevention. In *Behavioral health: A handbook of health enhancement and disease prevention*, ed. Matarazzo, J.D., Weiss, S.M., Herd, J.A. et al., 1171-1178. New York: John Wiley.

44. Solomon, D.S. and Maccoby, N. 1985. Communication as a model for health enhancement. In *Behavioral health: A handbook of health enhancement and disease prevention*, ed. Matarazzo, J.D., Weiss, S.M., Herd, J.A. et al., 209-221. New York: John Wiley.

45. Hunt, W.A., Barnett, L.W. and Branch, L.G. 1971. Relapse rates. *Journal of Clinical Psychology* 27:455-456.

Marlatt, G. and Gordon, J. 1985. *Relapse prevention: Maintenance strategies in the treatment of addictive behaviors.* New York: Guilford Press.

46. Wilson, G.T. 1985. Weight control treatments. In *Behavioral health: A handbook of health enhancement and disease prevention*, ed. Matarazzo, J.D., Weiss, S.M., Herd, J.A. et al., 657-670. New York: John Wiley.

47. Lichtenstein, E. and Mermelstein, R. 1985. Review of approaches to smoking treatment: Behavior modification strategies. In *Behavioral health: A handbook of health enhancement and disease prevention*, ed. Matarazzo, J.D., Weiss, S.M., Herd, J.A. et al., 695-712. New York: John Wiley.

48. Stall, R., Ekstrand, M., Pollack, M.L. et al. Forthcoming. Relapse from safe sex: The next challenge for AIDS prevention efforts. *Journal of AIDS.*

CHAPTER 4
A City Responds to Crisis: Creating New Approaches

1. Hessol, N.A., Lifson, A.R., O'Malley, P.M. et al. 1989. Prevalence, incidence and progression of human immunodeficiency virus infection in homosexual and bisexual men in hepatitis B vaccine trails, 1978-1988. *American Journal of Epidemiology* 130(6).

2. Rutherford, G.W. 1987. Testimony before the Human Resources and Intergovernmental Relations Subcommittee, U.S. House of Representatives, November.

3. San Francisco Department of Public Health, Office of AIDS. 1988. *AIDS in San Francisco: Status report for fiscal year 1987-88 and projections of service needs and costs for 1988-93*. These elements were first discussed at length in a report developed by the AIDS Office for the San Francisco Health Commission in March 1987. The report was updated and the discussion significantly expanded a year later.

4. San Francisco Department of Public Health, Office of AIDS. 1989. *AIDS Monthly Surveillance Report* (December 31). In each of the five years prior to 1986, homosexual or bisexual men comprised over 90 percent of the injection drug users diagnosed with AIDS in San Francisco.

5. See note 4 above.

6. See note 4 above.

CHAPTER 5
San Francisco's Prevention Partnership: Issues and Challenges

1. Imagawa, D.T., Lee, M.H., Wolinsky, S.M. et al. 1989. Human immunodeficiency virus type 1 infection in homosexual men who remain seronegative for prolonged periods. *The New England Journal of Medicine* 320(22): 1458-1462.

2. Lemp, G., Payne, S.F., Neal, D. et al. Survival trends for patients with AIDS. *Journal of the American Medical Association* 263(3): 405.

3. Udall, L. 1990. Personal communication, San Francisco Department of Public Health, Office of AIDS, March.

4. Amory, J.W. 1987. Personal communication to Congresswoman Nancy Pelosi, July. Some of the data from this letter were incorporated into a poster presentation at the 4th International Conference on AIDS.

    Woo, J.M., Neal, D.P., Geoghehan, C.M. et al. 1988. Evaluation of heterosexual contact tracing of partners of AIDS patients, poster presentation, 4th International Conference on AIDS, Stockholm.

5. Amory, J. 1988. Presentation before the San Francisco Health Commission, August 4.

6. See note 5 above.

7. San Francisco Department of Public Health, Office of AIDS. 1989. *AIDS Monthly Surveillance Report* (December 31). As of 12/31/89, 85 percent of the reported AIDS cases in the city's racial/ethnic minority communities are among homosexual or bisexual men; the range extends from 78 percent of Black cases to 91 percent of Hispanic cases.

CHAPTER 6
Lessons from San Francisco: Principles of Program Design

1. Research and Decisions Corporation. 1984. *Designing an effective AIDS prevention campaign strategy for San Francisco: Results from the first probability sample of an urban gay White male community*. San Francisco.

2. Stall, R. and Paul, J. 1989. Changes in sexual risk for infection with the human immunodeficiency virus among gay and bisexual men in San Francisco. Report to the World Health Organization Global Programme on AIDS, Geneva.

3. Stall, R., Ekstrand, M., Pollack, L. et al. Forthcoming. Relapse from safer sex: The next challenge for AIDS prevention efforts. *Journal of AIDS*.

4. Communication Technologies. 1988. Planning for the AIDS epidemic in California: A population-based assessment of knowledge, attitudes and behaviors. Report prepared for the State of California Department of Health Services, Office of AIDS, Sacramento, California.

CHAPTER 7
Planning and Implementing Community Strategies

1. Centers for Disease Control. 1982. *Morbidity and Mortality Weekly Report* 31 (September 24): 507-514.

2. Centers for Disease Control. 1990. *HIV/AIDS Surveillance Report* (January): 5.

3. See note 2 above.

4. Kubler-Ross, E. 1987. *AIDS: The ultimate challenge*, 1-2. New York: Macmillan.

5. Deaver, G.E.A. 1980. *Community health analysis*, 41-72. Germantown, MD: Aspen Systems.

The planning concepts described are drawn from Jantsch, E., 1972. *Technological planning and social futures*. London: Associated Business Programs.

6. National Academy of Sciences. 1989. *AIDS, sexual behavior, and intravenous drug use*, 317-318. Washington, DC.

Contributors

Jeffery W. Amory is a management consultant in private practice. He is former director of the AIDS Office of the San Francisco Department of Public Health.

Henrik L. Blum, MD, MPH, is Professor Emeritus of Health Policy and Planning at the University of California, Berkeley. He is the author of *Planning for Health* (Human Sciences Press, 1989) and *Expanding Health Care Horizons* (Third Party Publishing Company, 1989).

Margaret A. Chesney, PhD, is an Adjunct Professor in the Department of Epidemiology and Biostatistics at the University of California, San Francisco, and is affiliated with the Center for AIDS Prevention Studies of the University of California, San Francisco. She has contributed to *Women & AIDS: Promoting Healthy Behaviors* (U.S. Government Printing Office, In Press).

Pat Christen is Executive Director of the San Francisco AIDS Foundation. She has been with the Foundation since 1985, serving as the Media Relations Officer, Hotline Coordinator and Public Policy Director. Ms. Christen has written, studied and lectured on the subject of AIDS, both in this country and abroad.

Thomas J. Coates, PhD, is Associate Professor of Medicine and Director of Behavioral Medicine, Division of General Internal Medicine, at the University of California, San Francisco. He is Codirector of the Center for AIDS Prevention Studies of the University of California, San Francisco.

Pat Franks is a health policy analyst at the Institute for Health Policy Studies, University of California, San Francisco. She is also affiliated with the Center for AIDS Prevention Studies. She has provided technical assistance on HIV-related policies, programs and planning to the National Commission on AIDS, as well as to federal, state and local government and community-based agencies. Ms. Franks is coauthor of a number of books, reports and articles on health promotion and disease prevention and on AIDS.

Chuck Frutchey is Coeducation Director of the San Francisco AIDS Foundation and has been active in HIV education and prevention since 1982. Mr. Frutchey contributed to *AIDS: Principles, Practices and Politics* (Hemisphere Publishing Corporation, 1988) and *Promoting Safer Sex* (Swets and Zeitlinger, 1990).

Mindy Thompson Fullilove, MD, is Principal Investigator, Substance Abuse Core, at the HIV Center for Clinical and Behavioral Studies, New York City. She is former Director of Multicultural Inquiry and Research on AIDS, a program of the Bayview-Hunter's Point Foundation and the Center for AIDS Prevention Studies of the University of California, San Francisco.

Paul M. Gibson, LCSW, is HIV Prevention Coordinator, Division of STD Control, San Francisco Department of Public Health. He has written articles on the risk of HIV in youth and on HIV prevention for families with members at risk for infection. Mr. Gibson is affiliated with the AIDS Health Project of the University of California, San Francisco, as a group facilitator and referral therapist.

Joseph R. Guydish, PhD, is a Fellow at the Center for AIDS Prevention Studies of the University of California, San Francisco. He has written on risk behavior and behavior change among injection drug users.

Katherine C. Haynes, MBA, is Communications Director of Multicultural Inquiry and Research on AIDS, a program of the Bayview-Hunter's Point Foundation and the Center for AIDS Prevention Studies of the University of California, San Francisco. She has researched deaths from AIDS among Blacks and Latinos in the San Francisco Bay Area.

Stephen B. Hulley, MD, MPH, is Professor and Vice Chair of the Department of Epidemiology and Biostatistics at the University of California, San Francisco. He is also a Principal Investigator and Director at the Center for AIDS Prevention Studies of the University of California, San Francisco. He has written extensively on the epidemiology and prevention of HIV and other diseases and is the author of *Designing Clinical Research* (Williams and Wilkins, 1988).

Renata G. Kiefer, MD, a pediatrician and epidemiologist, is a Fellow at the Center for AIDS Prevention Studies of the University of California, San Francisco. She has served as a consultant on HIV policy in several countries, including Paraguay, and her writing includes articles on the cost-effectiveness of HIV screening in newborns.

George F. Lemp, MD, MPH, is Chief, Surveillance Branch, of the AIDS Office of the San Francisco Department of Public Health. His research and writing on HIV includes studies of survival trends for people with AIDS and projections of AIDS morbidity and mortality in San Francisco. Dr. Lemp has been a frequent presenter at annual sessions of the International Conference on AIDS.

Edward S. Morales, PhD, is an Assistant Professor at the California School of Professional Psychology, Berkeley. He was a founder of both the AIDS Health Project of the University of California, San Francisco, and Multicultural Inquiry and Research on AIDS, a program of the Bayview-Hunter's Point Foundation and the Center for AIDS Prevention Studies of the University of California, San Francisco.

Steven Petrow, a consulting editor and HIV educator, is author of *Dancing Against the Darkness: A Journey through America in the Age of AIDS* (Lexington Books, 1990). For five years, Mr. Petrow was a staff member and volunteer at the San Francisco AIDS Foundation. His writings about AIDS have appeared in the *Los Angeles Times*, the Los Angeles *Herald-Examiner*, and *The Advocate*. He currently serves as a member of the Alameda County AIDS Advisory Board.

Mervyn F. Silverman, MD, MPH, is President of the American Foundation for AIDS Research and Director of the Robert Wood Johnson Foundation AIDS Health Services Program. He is also Senior Technical Advisor to the AIDSCOM project of the Academy for Educational Development. Dr. Silverman is former Director of the San Francisco Department of Public Health.

Ron Stall, PhD, is an Assistant Adjunct Professor at the University of California, San Francisco, and is affiliated with the Center for AIDS Prevention Studies of the University of California, San Francisco. He has written on the association between drug and alcohol use and HIV, and on relapse from safe sex and is a principal of research on the epidemiology of AIDS among older Americans.

Timothy R. Wolfred, PsyD, a management consultant to human services programs, is former Executive Director of the San Francisco AIDS Foundation. He is a member of the Mayor's HIV Task Force in San Francisco. He currently serves as President of the Board of Governors of the San Francisco Community College District.